STRANGE TRIPS

MCGILL-QUEEN'S/ASSOCIATED MEDICAL SERVICES STUDIES
IN THE HISTORY OF MEDICINE, HEALTH, AND SOCIETY
SERIES EDITORS: J.T.H. CONNOR AND ERIKA DYCK

This series presents books in the history of medicine, health studies, and social policy, exploring interactions between the institutions, ideas, and practices of medicine and those of society as a whole. To begin to understand these complex relationships and their history is a vital step to ensuring the protection of a fundamental human right: the right to health. Volumes in this series have received financial support to assist publication from Associated Medical Services, Inc. (AMS), a Canadian charitable organization with an impressive history as a catalyst for change in Canadian healthcare. For eighty years, AMS has had a profound impact through its support of the history of medicine and the education of healthcare professionals, and by making strategic investments to address critical issues in our healthcare system. AMS has funded eight chairs in the history of medicine across Canada, is a primary sponsor of many of the country's history of medicine and nursing organizations, and offers fellowships and grants through the AMS History of Medicine and Healthcare Program (www.amshealthcare.ca).

STRANGE TRIPS

Science, Culture, and the Regulation of Drugs

LUCAS RICHERT

McGill-Queen's University Press
Montreal & Kingston • London • Chicago

© McGill-Queen's University Press 2018

ISBN 978-0-7735-5637-9 (cloth)
ISBN 978-0-7735-5652-2 (ePDF)
ISBN 978-0-7735-5653-9 (ePUB)

Legal deposit first quarter 2019
Bibliothèque nationale du Québec

Printed in Canada on acid-free paper that is 100% ancient forest free
(100% post-consumer recycled), processed chlorine free

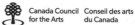

We acknowledge the support of the Canada Council for the Arts, which last year
invested $153 million to bring the arts to Canadians throughout the country.

Nous remercions le Conseil des arts du Canada de son soutien. L'an dernier,
le Conseil a investi 153 millions de dollars pour mettre de l'art dans la vie des
Canadiennes et des Canadiens de tout le pays.

Library and Archives Canada Cataloguing in Publication

Richert, Lucas, 1979–, author
Strange trips : science, culture, and the regulation of drugs / Lucas Richert.

(McGill-Queen's/Associated Medical Services studies in the history of medicine,
health, and society ; 51)
Includes bibliographical references and index.
Issued in print and electronic formats.
ISBN 978-0-7735-5637-9 (cloth). –ISBN 978-0-7735-5652-2 (ePDF). –
ISBN 978-0-7735-5653-9 (ePUB)

1. Drugs–Canada. 2. Drugs of abuse–Canada. 3. Drugs–United States.
4. Drugs of abuse–United States. I. Title. II. Series: McGill-Queen's/Associated
Medical Services studies in the history of medicine, health, and society ; 51
RM316.R53 2019   615.1   C2018-905685-1
                                       C2018-905686-x

This book was typeset in 10.5/13 Sabon.

For Meredith, who left us far too early

CONTENTS

ACKNOWLEDGMENTS

Marvellous communities of scholars and friends were supportive as I progressed through the ups and downs of this project. Special thanks to members of the Centre for the Social History of Health and Healthcare, University of Strathclyde. I've been surrounded by a superb collection of comrades, including Ved Baruah, Patricia Barton, Mark Ellis, Laura Kelly, Arthur McIvor, Emma Newlands, and Elsa Richardson. At CSHHH, Caroline Marley has brought a measure of order to the chaos and helped us unleash our potential. The support team in the School of Humanities has been stellar, too, and must be acknowledged for everything they have done for me during my time at Strathclyde. Very special thanks to Jim Mills, who has been an energetic and encouraging mentor. Matt Smith, an outstanding academic and a good friend, was also instrumental in the completion of this book.

The willingness of many scholars to share their time and ideas was incredibly important in the development of this project. While at the University of Saskatchewan, I was fortunate to work within a first-rate history of medicine research cluster, led by CRC Erika Dyck, who acted as collaborator, mentor, and friend. Her expertise and collaborative spirit were vital in the construction of chapter 4. Parts of this chapter were conceived and written in partnership with her, versions of which later appeared in *Plant Medicines, Healing and Psychedelic Science: Cultural Perspectives*, edited by Beatrix Caiuby Labate and Clancy Cavnar (Springer, 2018). Others who read and commented on this work to varying degrees include Mark Haden, Greg Higby, Stephen Parkin, and Percy Walton. Finally, thanks to a wide range of people who have been helpful along the rutted road, including: Virginia Berridge, William Booth, Nancy Campbell, Dorian Deshauer, Claire Clark, Jackie Duffin, Emily Dufton, Matthew Dziennik, W. Scott Haine, Jim Handy, David Herzberg, Timothy Hickman, Chris Hoff, Jackie Kripki, Emma Long, Dan Malleck, Sarah Marks, Helen Mawdsley, Stephen Mawdsley, Joe Merton, Adam Montgomery, Matthew Neufeld, Dan Peart, Nic Rasmussen, Mat Savelli, Phillip Smith, Joe Spillane, Jon Sutton, Richard Warden, Cheryl Krasnick Warsh, and Manuela Williams. At MQUP, Kyla Madden and the production team have been terrific. Recognition, of course, must be given to my external reviewers and copy editors for taking the time to read and make useful suggestions to improve the manuscript. Finally, thanks to Matthew DeCloedt, a superb research associate and friend.

This project would not have been possible without the generous support of various institutions, organizations, and archives. Archival gatekeepers Diana Bachman, Jessica Borge, Sam Maddra, and Sarah Hepworth were crucial. I'm certain to miss someone, so please forgive me. I must also thank the Wellcome Trust and the Social Science and Humanities Research Council of Canada for funding me several years ago, as well as convey gratitude to the Canadian Association for the History of Medicine and American Association for the History of Medicine. Early versions of this work appeared in the pages of the *Canadian Review of American Studies* and *Pharmacy in History*.

This book begins with a dedication to my mother, Meredith. She struggled with different forms of cancer and tried several strange medicines during her losing battle. As an undergraduate student in my early twenties, I had no idea then that the experience would lead me on this pathway. Thanks to my other family members who have listened to my stories about drugs and medicines, and the peculiar line that separated them. You know who you are.

Lastly, thank you to my wife Elizabeth for being my best friend, as well as to my luminescent children, Oscar and Lucy, who are generous with their light.

STRANGE TRIPS

INTRODUCTION:
BEYOND SUBSTANCES IN SILOS

Drugs. Pharmaceuticals. Intoxicants. Substances. Medicines. Each word has been invested with degrees of legitimacy and illegitimacy, as well as legality and illegality. And these words have always correlated with consumption, control, and political agendas. In recent years, both recreational and pharmaceutical drugs have seized the general public's attention for numerous reasons. Whether it is the modification of marijuana laws in the United States and Canada, a dreadful opioid crisis, or the ongoing discussions about the elevating costs of legitimate products in the US (think of the cartoonish villain Martin Shkreli and Mylan's EpiPen prices), the public's awareness of drugs has grown more acute. An increasing number of US states have passed medical marijuana legislation, whereas the Canadian government, led by the Justin Trudeau Liberals, initiated full-on legalization efforts in 2015. Recent TV series and major motion pictures such as *Breaking Bad*, *House M.D.*, *Narcos*, and *Sicario* have featured stories reducible to illicit drug manufacture and use, the regulation of pharmaceuticals, and, yes, a monolithically greedy drug industry. The wonderful surprise hit of 2016, *Stranger Things*, featured a telekinetic and telepathic girl whose superpowers derived from a mother who had undergone unsanctioned LSD experiments in a shady government facility. Additionally, it is impossible to turn on the evening news without hearing about drugs, and the importance of drugs in contemporary life. One does not need to think any further than the ongoing opioid crisis gripping Canada and the United States.

Since World War II, government, industry, and academia have demonstrated a mixed record in framing policies and generating knowledge to address drug use and misuse, both within and outside the medical realm. New studies have sought to understand the rise of drug regulation through different prisms, whether the vestiges of capitalism, liberalism, or a case study of the Bureau of Narcotics.[1] Others have gone further back. "The use of intoxicating substances has been a perennial aspect of human history," Michele Rotunda argued in 2007, "even as the manner in which it has been understood and interpreted has changed."[2] For her, thinking historically about how and why the overuse of certain intoxicating substances was construed as a specific disease, or simply demonized for that matter, offers a window into the relationship between scientific knowledge, cultural assumptions, and social concerns. A failure to recognize this clouds the policy-making process, and some commentators have archly diagnosed this problem as "Drug Policy Abuse," essentially a condition preventing elected officials and public figures from producing rational decisions about drugs, be they prescription painkillers or fake fentanyl purchased at a nightclub.[3] The symptoms of this abusive behaviour often include an unwillingness to talk openly about drugs, a failure to recognize the determinants involved in drug misuse, and an inability to examine the available evidence.

Governments and medical authorities must reflect on consumer protection and drug regulation, commercial considerations, and their responsibility to guard citizens from unauthorized businesses, including dispensaries and head shops. *Strange Trips* can play a part in this drama. Whether the topic is access to heroin or Laetrile in the treatment of cancer, medical marijuana in Canada, or LSD for death and depression, there is always room for more information, including a historical perspective. This book will investigate the myths, meanings, and boundaries of certain recreational drugs and pharmaceuticals. It will unpack how we have regarded and regulated drugs in light of long-standing economic and political interests related to medicine, be they companies or professional bodies. Scholars have, to date, focused on a host of substances, from coffee to wine through to nicotine, opium, and even chocolate. In short, we have exposed important biographies of substances. Yet, in 2017, historian Virginia Berridge, while giving a keynote address before the Alcohol and Drugs History Society in Utrecht, called for a *move beyond* examining substances in silos.

This book is, in part, a reply to that call. It puts drugs in conversation with each other. *Strange Trips* examines control and resistance in palliative care drugs, recreational drugs, and pharmaceutical drugs. What, I wonder, is the path that a drug such as heroin takes in its move from radical and illegal drug to an accepted part of medical practice? Is it the same course that LSD or Laetrile might chart? Conversely, how do accepted pills, manufactured in the US by respectable companies such as Pfizer or Merck, become characterized as dangerous, even radical? In addressing such questions in a broad fashion, we can begin to see links between money and bodies, politics and personal choice. By retracing some of this recent history, *Strange Trips* can provide a more expansive view, or an interpretation that has ramifications for law and medicine. This might, in turn, permit a bird's-eye view into the role that various companies and institutions play in creating medical knowledge and ideas about our bodies – in other words, everyday health. Facts about drugs and medicine change, but often this story is left untold.* When policies are made, votes cast, and prescriptions written, it is useful to have a deeper sense of how the "facts" are fluid.

Other writers have suggested we need to enhance the "evidence about evidence" when it comes to drugs, science, and policy.[4] For Alan Leshner, former head of the National Institute of Drug Abuse and member of the US National Science Board, "there is a unique disconnect between the scientific facts and the public's perception about drug abuse and addiction."[5] Or, as the British psychopharmacologist David Nutt has put it, emphasis ought to be placed on "evidence, not exaggeration," making it time to reconsider *Drugs without the Hot Air*, the title of his 2012 book. He suggested that Ecstasy was "no more dangerous than horse riding," and afterward was fired as the British government's chief drug advisor when he stated that alcohol and tobacco were more harmful than many illegal drugs, including LSD, Ecstasy, and cannabis. Nutt continued his neurological and psychiatric research at Imperial College London and argued through the BBC and *The Guardian* that magic mushrooms, LSD, Ecstasy, cannabis, and mephedrone all possessed therapeutic applications. He was (and still is) a central figure in the understanding of so-called recreational (or street) drugs and

---

* One trip that this book won't deal with, however, is the World Trade Organization's (WTO) Trade-Related Aspects of Intellectual Property Rights Agreement (otherwise known as the TRIPS agreement). It established the minimum standards for protection of intellectual property; these include patents for pharmaceuticals. TRIPS has been critiqued because it has been shown to increase drug prices.

legitimate medical therapies. His agenda is clear. "I'm not recommending anyone taking any drugs," he stated. "I'm just suggesting we need to have a more scientific rational approach to drugs."[6]

In *Strange Trips*, it will become abundantly clear that it is time to move beyond the pharmaceutical industry (sometimes called Big Pharma) and the Food and Drug Administration (FDA) in exploring drugs in the twenty-first century. It is time to seek a firmer grasp of the complex boundaries among legal and recreational drugs, the back-and-forth struggles over acceptance and illegality in the realms of science, as well as the debates in the media and political sphere.[7] With my first book, *Conservatism, Consumer Choice, and the Food and Drug Administration during the Reagan Era: A Prescription for Scandal*, I examined the political, economic, and social aspects of pharmaceuticals in the United States from the 1970s to the 1990s. Product innovation, consumer protection, and freedom of choice in the medical marketplace were complicated by competing ideologies and principles. Also muddying matters were the rise of potent health activist groups, including HIV/AIDS activists, and strong institutional forces within the FDA. Occasionally, scandal and controversy – even tragedy – resulted from the anti-regulatory ethos of the mid-1980s, or from pharmaceutical industry practices. In other instances, health activists, politicians, and FDA regulators demonstrated policy innovation and tackled major health problems with a mixture of originality and courage.

Through the topic of strange medicines it is possible to facilitate a more complete picture of how medical knowledge has been established and codified, treatments developed, and medicines legitimized. Alternatives may appear and disappear as mainstream medicine selects, refines, or rejects them; new alternatives are constantly generated by the limitations and weaknesses of the elite practices they run alongside. Insights from Collins and Pinch's *Dr. Golem*, for example, focus on the perennial tension between "science and succor," or the struggle between well-regarded, evidence-based therapies and the psychic needs of the patient.[8] In *Dr. Golem*, we witness a vital historical contradiction in patient-consumer agency. For scientists and medical practitioners, wisdom dictates that therapies be predicated on collective judgment about the best scientific evidence. Yet, for patients and caregivers, more benefits may come from a sympathetic human exchange between healer and patient, as well as the fact that hope matters. And hope often lies in a roll of the dice rather than a treatment based on frequently dismal probabilities of scientific protocols. Evidence matters less, which raises several questions. Based on the best practices, what medicines ought to be consumed at the end of life? For patients and caregivers, do such therapies meet their needs? In *Strange Trips*, we will see that answers to such inquiries are far from clear.

PILLARS OF THE BOOK

Debates about the salience and suitability of drugs in medical practice do not occur in a vacuum. As such, there are some pillars to keep in mind when reading my book.

First, as various governments of different political stripes have sought to limit the volume and use of recreational drugs in the US and Canada, pharmaceutical products and advertisements have grown more ubiquitous in everyday life. A "big and bold" war on drugs has proceeded since the early 1970s, costing hundreds of billions of dollars. In the United States, President Nixon launched the first drug war following the conclusion of the 1960s. Following the passage of the Comprehensive Drug Abuse and Prevention Control Act of 1970, in June of 1971, Nixon officially declared a War on Drugs and called drug abuse "enemy number one in America."[9] That same year, Nixon created the Special Action Office for Drug Abuse Prevention (SAODAP) within the Executive Office of the President as a "dramatic way to highlight the problem."[10]

Then, President Ronald Reagan initiated his massive War on Drugs. It included the Anti-Drug Abuse Act of 1986, crack cocaine rhetoric, a "Just Say No" campaign, and Public Service Announcements, featuring Clint Eastwood, Mel Gibson, Pee Wee Herman, and the indomitable Mr. T.[11] Nancy Reagan served as the point person. By 1989, she had given more than 1,200 interviews, delivered 49 speeches, inspired 12,000 "Just Say No" clubs, and motivated more than five million people to show up to "Just Say No" marches in 700 cities.[12] Interestingly, pharmaceutical companies from the early 1980s emerged at this time as incomparable titans of industry. As I conceived of my first book, *A Prescription for Scandal*, I found this a fascinating historical phenomenon and one I wanted to explore further; thus, the following pages examine the struggle between established pharmaceutical companies and peripheral products struggling for validity, whether the product happened to be heroin, cannabis, or LSD. Were these contested medicines patentable and economically viable, or did they represent additional – and unwanted – competition in the medical marketplace? This idea pops up early and often.

Second, historians of drugs have long held a view that substances have specific careers. These careers have usually involved intense periods of enthusiasm, therapeutic optimism, critical appraisals, and eventually limited use.[13] The careers of drugs in modern medicine are also driven by various factors, including biomedical research, marketing, and industry and consumer demands. Often, the conclusion has been that drugs – whether they be LSD or heroin or ketamine – circulate through consistent patterns and in due course wane into disuse. Sometimes they can make a comeback. Sometimes the cycle concludes with the total disappearance of the drug from health care, only to be replaced by newer – and better – versions ready to follow similar careers. But a drug can of course also reappear and start a new career cycle, for instance on the introduction of a different diagnostic disorder, or for other cultural, medical, or economic reasons. The 1960s and 1970s, for instance, witnessed a countercultural revolution that swept the United States and Canada, and, at least in the former, undermined the love affair with scientific and medical expertise. More alternative health books appeared. The cachet associated with natural medicines increased. Understanding one's body and health became a statement of self-determination.[14] Now, while the length of time for a drug cycle differs, depending on contextual factors, the overall model remains a useful one for considering the life cycle of a drug. As Pieters and Snelders described it in 2007:

> The medical market is made receptive by a growing number of favourable scientific reports, positive discussions of the new drug by influential members of the medical profession and coverage in the media. A wave of public enthusiasm makes the drug fashionable. Growing use of the drug and high expectations of its therapeutic effects are usually followed by a negative reaction when it does not live up to its exaggerated reputation.[15]

To put this more simply, the popularity and use of drugs ebbs and flows. Drugs journey across the blurry line of legality and illegality, acceptance and demonization. The specific framework in which the scientific evidence is produced plays a significant role in how the drug is assessed, and the extent to which it is considered novel. Together, medico-scientific, economic, and socio-cultural factors shape the career cycles and should not be understated.*[16]

Third, and related to the second pillar, is evidence. With both recreational drugs and pharmaceutical products, all of the users and regulators, physicians, researchers, and law enforcement officials, must negotiate how *evidence shapes a given policy*. Debates recur about whether policies are actually *based* on evidence, or are merely *informed* by it.[17] Ultimately, whatever one believes on this score, a "consumer protection" model often runs up against a "social control" model as proponents of each evaluate the evidence, usually scientific studies.[18] Here, medical and scientific knowledge of medicines is disputed; and one can also detect the broader tensions between consumer choice and the state's obligation to offer protections for its people. To what extent, in short, should government limit and control access to drugs? What are the boundaries of legitimate and illegitimate use in the laboratory and on the street? What is the proper balance between research and development and consumer protection?[19] Answering these questions is no simple task, especially when, according to the book *Buzzed*, most interpretations of the scientific literature relevant to drugs such as heroin or LSD are "oversimplified, inaccurate, or disseminated by organizations that slant the research to further political and moral agendas."[20] As the editors of *Scientific American* suggest, LSD serves as a prime example of how "hyperbolic rhetoric that is a legacy of the war on drugs" has negatively influenced basic science and, ultimately, hampered our ability to manage reactions to these drugs.[21]

Fourth, alcohol and tobacco do not operate in a separate realm from more radical drugs or pharmaceuticals. So-called "normalized" drugs – booze and cigarettes – also have highly contested histories and have

---

* Racial categories, for instance, are important in the ways intoxicants, medicines, and regulations are regarded. Nunn (423) suggests that we "must recognize the central role drug trafficking has played in the European conquest of other cultures and the maintenance of white supremacy worldwide." Addictive and deleterious substances were used to undermine non-European societies and further white interests, weakening a country or culture internally – as well as limiting its ability to resist white economic or cultural intrusion. Drug laws themselves have often been regarded as a means to control certain ethnic groups, although historians such as Dan Malleck have pushed back against this line of reasoning. Ethnicity and race are not major features of this book, but are certainly worth bearing in mind.

been subject to cycles of optimism and acceptance, disenchantment and bans. Alcohol was once deeply embedded in North American culture, institutionalized in religious, medical, military, and political practices. Yet, broad-based social movements at the turn of the century forced its prohibition, driving US alcohol underground from 1920 to 1933.[22] Similarly, tobacco was a drug that defined North America, particularly the United States. Just as alcohol was used as a medicine, tobacco once had an assigned therapeutic value. Europeans who arrived in North America found that Indigenous peoples used tobacco for a variety of spiritual, social, and medicinal healing purposes. Thereafter, European settlers experimented with the drug, recording a number of physiological effects. Cigarettes, which would later become a staple part of North American economies, were employed for curing coughs as well as staying trim. According to historian Allan Brandt in *The Cigarette Century*, tobacco companies cleverly sought to reassure the public of the competitive health advantages of their brands, recruit physicians as crucial allies in the ongoing process of marketing tobacco, and vigorously contest categorical scientific findings about the negative health effects of smoking. In the realm of pharmaceuticals, historians David Herzberg and Jeremy Greene are driving new analyses of the use and misuse of pharmaceuticals, and the ways in which companies marketed addictive prescription drugs to patient-consumers.[23]

Crucially, in a number of the following chapters, these kinds of actions play out again and again. David Michaels, a public health writer, has characterized obstructionism on the part of pharmaceutical companies as attempts to "manufacture uncertainty" about the claims of danger about their products and thereby delay regulatory action. Just like Big Tobacco fought scientific findings, Big Pharma resists negative claims about their products. Michaels writes, "with study after study, year after year. Data are disputed, data have to be reanalyzed. More research is always needed. Uncertainty is manufactured."[24] While this book does not examine alcohol or tobacco, it's worthwhile being aware of these other contested substances. It's beneficial to recognize that substances, as much as they are distinct, also have shared histories.

Finally, as the data over trippy drugs are analyzed and reanalyzed, discussions persist about *taking literal trips* to obtain different kinds of drugs. Medical tourism, the last pillar of this book, has its origins in ancient times, when the sick and spiritual alike visited holy sites, mineral waters, or healing temples such as the Temple of Delphi. Today international medical tourism has blossomed in Asia, India, and elsewhere, raising major questions about patient choice and access to services, as well as other unintended consequences of globalized medicine. On the one hand, some appraisals hold medical tourism as *widening* health disparities, even as the quality of the health care in destination countries is challenged. On the other hand, supporters submit that tourism helps lower in-country health care costs and promotes development, while acting as a means to fund existing services – basically, a leveller of inequality.[25] Either way, patients have adopted medical tourism to get their hands on drugs and new medical treatments. At the beginning of the 1980s, actor Steve McQueen searched desperately for hope in his struggle against cancer. He found it, along with unapproved and experimental drugs, as well as a bizarre array of other therapies, in Mexico. Another example is cross-border pharmaceutical purchasing. In Canada, the federal government regulates drug prices, and by the mid-1990s plenty of Americans found great bargains in their friendly neighbour across the 49th parallel. All of this changed, though, after September 11, 2001, when pharmaceutical products sold in Canada – either online or in person – were demonized as harshly as any other street drug, whether it be smack or crack. Even more recently, Canadian citizens suffering from treatment-resistant depression have travelled to the United States for experimental ketamine therapy. In short, it will become clear throughout this book that patients have, at various times, taken trips to get hold of strange and not-so-strange medicines.

BOOK DESIGN: BLUEPRINT

The following chapters investigate the histories of pharmaceuticals and recreational drugs from diverse perspectives. But this book is not theory-driven. The aim isn't to prove any of my colleagues right or wrong. Each chapter, to varying degrees, reflects who was representative of capitalistic tendencies in medicine, medical tourism, and choice – as well as exploring the use of alternative approaches and competing medical knowledge. The following chapters examine science, the pharmaceutical industry, and cultural artifacts. Instead of a discrete and exclusive focus on a single substance such as cocaine or a specific class of drugs such as SSRIs, this book illustrates several

overlapping stories. It studies several drug careers to remove substances from their silos. I will clarify competing medical knowledges
(and counter-knowledges). I will unpick orthodox and alternative
narratives, with all of the related conspiratorial and mainstream
undercurrents. Scientific consensus on a given medicine fluctuates
over time, if it ever existed at all; facts and fiction are distorted and
citizens are occasionally left scratching their heads. People may feel
they have been hoodwinked by pharmaceutical companies into consuming dangerous products, or, slightly less bad, have been swindled
into paying exorbitant prices. Additionally, people may feel that there
are better options available in the medical marketplace, and that the
government or the medical community has no right to deny access
to strange medicines, such as heroin or LSD or cannabis. The following pages will recount stories like these, potentially act as a reference
point, and add historical layers to contemporary discussions.

Geographically, this book will concentrate on Canada and the
United States, sometimes independently, and sometimes as the countries negotiated with each other. At times, policies diverged; at other
moments, policies converged. I will not offer a direct comparative
analysis between the two countries, but will at times flag similarities
and differences. Temporally, the bulk of the book will be set during
the late 1960s and 1970s to the present. By no means is this a hard-
and-fast rule, though. It will become clear that the book occasionally
extends further back than the 1960s to pull on earlier strings. I leave
to future scholars deeper and discrete biographies of substances
and more reflective histories of healers, shamans, and the *dramatis
personae* influencing drug policy. Regional and religious histories of
drugs also warrant their own studies.

In the course of this book, I'll occasionally draw on popular culture, be it major films, fiction, or television, so that I may point out
useful connections and demonstrate not just how drugs have shaped
human society, but how pop culture has reflected back and given
shape to drugs and medicines. While I may not be a cultural historian per se, I do not agree with the contention that it is risky to
deduce politics from movies and music. To understand drugs in the
1960s, 1970s, and beyond, it is vital to have at least some sense
of fluffy cultural relics such as bell-bottoms, disco, and shag car-
pet.[26] Even more, it is critical to place regulatory initiatives like the
War on Drugs alongside such films as *Easy Rider* (1969) or *The
French Connection* (1971). The following history will not proceed

in a uniformly chronological fashion, nor will it employ linear argu-
mentation. Instead, the narrative hangs together by interwoven drug
stories. The pillars mentioned above spiral and circulate both hor-
izontally and vertically. Cultural references intersect with government documents, magazine coverage, medical journals, and so on.

Overall, I will place a spotlight on the process by which a drug may
move into the realm of the legitimate medical marketplace, or conversely how it may be cast out. The goal is to furnish an appreciation
of how substances have been demonized or rejuvenated, banned or
unshackled. I believe this is crucial, because challenging the multiple
myths and meanings behind drugs also supplements timely public discussions, pushes current historical views of various drugs in new directions, and transcends partisan battle-lines to generate novel approaches
to public policy. The drugs in this book – the strange medicines – naturally provoke different responses, and from all sorts of socio-political
and economic venues. They raise questions about scientific authority
and the production of medical knowledge, liberty, and collective goals
as a society. They conjure images of the pharmaceutical industry and
high costs. The spectre of prohibitionist impulses is called to mind. So
is quackery. Even more, therapeutic tools, whether they be ketamine,
cannabis, or Laetrile, have challenged the physician's influence over
patient-consumer choice in the medical marketplace.

The book is broken into three sections. The first, "End-of-Life
Medicines," centres on drugs in palliative care settings. Chapter 1
places a focus on heroin and its return to the medical marketplace in
Canada, specifically for pain management purposes in hospitals. In
the early 1980s, heroin emerged as a more humane solution for terminally ill cancer patients in Canada suffering tremendous amounts of
pain. As late as 1955, heroin was employed by physicians to alleviate
such pain, yet the stigma associated with the drug relegated it to the
sidelines of mainstream medical practice. With the publication of several American studies that found heroin to be superior to morphine
and the British health system's implementation of heroin treatment,
the cultural, medical, and political dispute in Canada began to inten-
sify throughout the early 1980s. Against the larger backdrop of the
American "War on Cancer" and "War on Drugs," heroin was debated
within the Canadian Medical Association and the federal government.
How, activists cried, could terminally ill cancer patients be denied a
powerful analgesic in the face of mounting evidence and political support? Why would palliative care doctors and the Canadian Cancer

Association be against it? Chapter 2 focuses on the contemporane-ous American discussion over heroin. What becomes clear is that the Canadian and American debates shared many attributes, including considerations about evidence, hesitancy on the part of elected offi-cials, the role of activists, and so forth; it's important to note that the American discussions were dissimilar for various reasons, including racial reasons. The role of African-American political leaders, includ-ing Charlie Rangel, helped define the American struggle. Soon the medical debate was politicized and overwhelmed by racial undertones.

Chapter 3 shifts away from heroin, but remains fixed on end-of-life therapies and the "correct" medicines to take at the terminus of one's fight with cancer. Indeed, individuals stricken with cancer had numerous strange medicines to choose from, one of which was called Laetrile, an unapproved product that can be found all over the globe in such foods as chickpeas, lentils, lima beans, cashews, et cetera. Promoted as a cancer treatment in the 1970s, Laetrile raised questions about the proper approach to terminally ill can-cer patients and the availability of certain "outsider" drugs. The debate over the use and availability of Laetrile mirrored many of the same ideas in the discussion over heroin, including consumer choice, government intrusion, and the availability of drugs in the medical marketplace. A key difference, though, was that heroin was to mitigate pain closer to the end of one's life, whereas Laetrile was promoted as a potential tool for actually saving one's life. While Laetrile had certainly been part of medical practice since at least the 1st–2nd century AD, it was bound up in the ascendance of alternative healing and holistic medicine during the 1960s, thereby increasing its use in the United States. From the Food and Drug Administration's perspective – which mattered, since it was the regulatory body governing the drug market in the US – only minimal anecdotal evidence supported the use of Laetrile. After an extensive five-month review, the agency argued there was insuf-ficient scientific proof to justify its use at all. The agency deemed it worthless and illegal as a cancer remedy. And yet, supporters viewed the FDA's ban on Laetrile as a restraint on individual free-dom. One of the notable individuals who epitomized freedom and coolness was actor Steve McQueen, who also struggled with cancer in the late 1970s and early 1980s. The medical profession largely derided his use of Laetrile in Mexico, but to some people with can-cer, McQueen's pursuit of an alternative treatment seemed heroic.

This chapter examines the life cycles of Laetrile, with particular attention paid to McQueen's role in this dispute.

The second section of the book is called "Hippy Medicine." And I don't mean this negatively. Chapter 4 showcases the debate about lysergic acid diethylamide (LSD) and highlights the political and socio-economic difficulties in breaching the barrier of drug legitimacy. This chapter demonstrates how physicians have employed LSD for mental illness and alcohol treatment, even as they faced resistance from the mainstream medical establishment and struggled with legality and claims about effectiveness and safety. Even more broadly, LSD – a strange medicine, for sure – provides a strong entry point into debates concerning how researchers and health professionals reacted to government claims about mind-altering drugs *and* the fluidity of what constitutes a "legitimate" versus a "recreational" drug. Moreover, through a study of LSD, Ecstasy, and ketamine as treatment modalities, one can interrogate the anti-drug rhetoric in the mid-1960s with contemporary discussion and form a nuanced historical perspective on psychiatry's approach to standard psychopharmaceuticals, such as Thorazine, Haldol, and Stelazine, drugs of the tranquilizer class.

In chapter 5, the subject is cannabis – specifically, cannabis in Canada. The thought of marijuana often conjures ideas of 1936's *Reefer Madness*, Harry J. Anslinger, or, later, Cheech and Chong's *Up in Smoke* and Bob Marley. In digging deeper than such basic references to pot in popular culture, one can appreciate a far more stimulating and complex story. In 2015, *The Economist* showcased the hazy future of Canadian recreational and medical pot and suggested that "converting a medical-marijuana industry into a recreational one will not be easy."[27] Many questions will have to be addressed and the transition could be rocky. As a Colorado marijuana enforcement official told the Canadian media, "It's going to be a lot harder to implement than you think. It's going to take a lot longer to do it. And it's going to cost more than you think."[28] The Liberal campaign promise of legalization has invited a new host of critics. John Ivison has reconceived Canada Post as Canada Pot, the major domestic system of distribution throughout the country. Sylvain Charlebois deems marijuana a "gateway" drug with high upsides. Dan Malleck has argued that liquor control boards should control recreational marijuana, whereas Lee Fang has argued persuasively that both the alcohol and pharmaceutical industries have sought to stymie the growth of the marijuana industry, a natural competitor. Money has always been a factor in the marijuana business. And many news alerts about marijuana in 2016–17 were not necessarily about seized cash or impounded product, but rather about stock offerings, business opportunities, and industry growth profiles.[29] This chapter will try to understand how cannabis has become more civilized in Canada.

The final section of the book, "Demonized Pharmaceuticals," spins the narrative in an alternative direction, as it underlines how drugs can be jolted from a position of acceptance and get rejected by medical and regulatory authorities, public officials, and consumers. Chapter 6, "The Maple Peril and the War on Terror: Pharmaceuticals in the Wake of September 11," examines the ways in which Canadian pharmaceutical products were demonized after the new millennium's first transformative moment, September 11, 2001. That year, the safety of drugs purchased from other countries, especially Canada, became a major policy issue in the United States. Approved drugs – in both the US and Canada – became a contentious issue. A political and geographical line was drawn in the sand, separating Canadian and American pills. In short, Canadian drugs were characterized as dangerous – essentially, "a maple peril." According to the health interest group Public Citizen, this was part of "the other drug war" in the United States. In this case, there were no crack babies or gun violence, and no "Just Say No" slogans or debates about rising rates of incarceration. Instead, the pharmaceutical industry and its drug representatives in the US Congress waged a different kind of war. As I explore the practice of cross-border drug reimportation and consider the Bush and Clinton administrations' policies regarding the necessary balance between drug access, affordability, and safety, it will become clear how Big Pharma in the US worked to demonize Canadian drugs in very crafty ways. It will also become clear that all sorts of medicines are contested in the modern medical marketplace, not simply radical or experimental drugs.

The book's penultimate chapter uses a recent and tragically pre-dictable period of drug history to examine obesity and quick-fix diet pills in the United States. North Americans, especially homemaker mothers and working-class women, have used cigarettes, amphet-amines, tapeworms, and an assortment of other products to maintain their figures over the years. In this chapter, the book will zero in on over-the-counter diet drugs containing phenylpropanolamine (PPA), a lesser-known kind of drug. In the early 1980s, such pills became a point of contestation among Congress, the FDA, and health watch-dog organizations. While some regulatory authorities had declared PPA safe, members of the US House of Representatives and activists in the Center for Science in the Public Interest claimed it was linked to hypertension, potentially fatal heart problems, kidney disease, and muscle damage. As one would expect, stakeholders fiercely negotiated with each over the intricacies of scientific data and, ultimately, their collective stories cast new light on the scourge of quick fixes and diet cures in contemporary society. By examining the clash over PPA diet pills from 1979 to 2000, I hope to contribute to a developing litera-ture on health, wellness, and "fatness" in the US.

Finally, the book ends with a ketamine conclusion, or coda. As became clear in the May 2017 issue of *The Lancet Psychiatry*, which had no fewer than five articles on ketamine, the drug has moved from the domain of dangerous product into a widely discussed tool.[30] Canadians are travelling to the United States for special treatments. Doctors on both sides of the border are questioning the drug's use. Maybe not a magic bullet yet, the drug is at least being discussed as a tool in the physician's black bag. This is why it's a useful means to bring an end to my analysis; the dialogue about ketamine exempli-fies how the public, the scientific community, and regulatory bodies in the US, Canada, and beyond grapple with the border separating licit and illicit drugs.

Part One

END-OF-LIFE
MEDICINE

MEDICAL HEROIN'S RETURN TO CANADA: PAIN, PALLIATIVE CARE, AND COLONIAL MEDICINE

In 2013–14, the rise of controversial heroin-assisted therapy in Vancouver generated heated policy discussions. While some Canadians were offended upon learning that physicians in Vancouver were administering pharmaceutical-grade heroin to addicts for maintenance and crime-prevention purposes, others regarded it as rational, evidence-based healthcare. Canada's federal health minister Rona Ambrose, who was strongly opposed to the practice, subsequently oversaw the passage of regulations in October 2013 that prevented any heroin-assisted therapy outside of limited clinical trials. This curtailed the treatment because it barred physicians from prescribing heroin to their patients, even when they thought it was the best treatment option available. Reaction was swift. The Pivot Legal Society, a group of lawyers representing the physicians and addicts, asserted that "ideology and not evidence" drove the health minister's decision, and that this decision put "the lives of heroin users at risk." Writing of the debate in *The Globe and Mail*, Peter McKnight argued, "drug laws have never been about improving health or reducing crime," and so in his estimation the attempt to ban heroin therapy was far from surprising.[1]

Health Canada's decision did not signal an end to the saga. In November 2014, five plaintiffs sought and won an injunction against Ambrose's regulation, which meant that 120 Vancouver-based addicts (who were deemed resistant to standard treatments) would be given pharmaceutical-grade heroin to minimize illicit drug use and criminal activity. It was a small victory for heroin-assisted therapy in Canada and a welcome affirmation for evidence-based harm reduction policies.

This episode in Vancouver was by no means the first discussion over the return of heroin (diamorphine) therapy in Canada. In the late 1970s and 1980s, medical, law enforcement, and political authorities came into conflict over its use as a humane solution for terminally ill cancer patients suffering through tremendous amounts of pain. The controlled legalization of heroin for the dying ultimately triggered an intricate, multifaceted, and revealing discussion about the political, economic, and cultural meanings of heroin in Canadian society. Such discussions were also ongoing in the United States and these prompted further reflections on individual pain in Canada. To what extent, legislators and physicians asked, should government limit access to heroin for the terminally ill? What was the proper balance between research, medical authority, and consumer protection for those patients who were suffering excruciating pain?[2] Heroin, in short, acted as a vehicle to examine drug history, the politics of pain management, and end-of-life policies in the 1970s and 1980s. It was another way in which parties in the medical marketplace, from physicians and regulators to drug industry representatives and health activists, contested the meanings and acceptance of medicines. According to Carnwath and White, "heroin is particularly good at inducing opinions which conflict with all the evidence and 'evidence' that is then moulded to fit the opinions."[3] This chapter explores the struggle over heroin as an accepted tool in the doctor's bag and exposes the contest over heroin as it sought to migrate from its position of illegitimacy in the medical marketplace.

The proposal for the legalization of heroin in Canada initially found opposition in the Liberal government of Canada and later with the Canadian Cancer Society. On the other side, with a national platform on which to make his case, nationally syndicated columnist W. Gifford-Jones soon gathered tremendous public support, as well as fellow champions in the Conservative Party and the Canadian Medical Association. "Never, never allow politicians to surround heroin use with red tape. If you accept this proviso you lose the game," Gifford-Jones said in an interview in 1989.[4] In the United States, where the debate was similarly in full swing, Gifford-Jones also had allies. "It is time," asserted Judith Quattlebaum, the founder of the US-based Committee for the Treatment for Intractable Pain (CTIP), "to give up our excessive fear of heroin ... Its legitimate use, when death is close, outweighs its total prohibition on grounds of abuse in any thoughtful ethical formulation."[5]

W. GIFFORD-JONES: CELEBRITY DOCTOR
AND HEROIN ADVOCATE

In 1979, a Toronto-based celebrity doctor and syndicated news-paper columnist, Kenneth Walker, who wrote under the pseud-onym W. Gifford-Jones, launched a campaign to legalize heroin in Canada and created a *cause célèbre*. In his estimation, heroin embodied one answer to the multifaceted problem of treating pain in Canadian society. Over a period of six years he raised close to a million dollars in support of his cause, even as he generated public and political awareness and faced resistance in the form of the Canadian Cancer Society, the Canadian Society of Hospi-tal Pharmacists, and the Royal Canadian Mounted Police. Walk-er's main platform was his column, called "The Doctor Game," printed in approximately ninety newspapers across the coun-try. Later, in 1983, after sparking parliamentary discussion and prompting thousands of letters from Canadians, Walker created the W. Gifford-Jones Foundation to solicit donations so that he could "continue the fight."[6] In charting his long struggles against the "establishment," Gifford-Jones would later position himself – rather improperly – alongside both Louis Pasteur and Ignaz Semmelweis.[7] In his autobiography, he noted that he was charac-terized as misinformed, headline-seeking, and radical, but that he valiantly resisted the "insurmountable" opposition.[8]

Walker initially launched the campaign in his January 1979 col-umn. His New Year's Eve resolution, he wrote, was to add heroin to the list of legitimate painkillers in Canada, and little did he realize that it would open "Pandora's box" and embroil him in such "con-troversy."[9] He offered a short history of heroin, outlined the "merits" of the drug, and described its use in the UK. As he put it, Canadians were denied heroin because of "political, not medical, decisions."[10]

Canada's most crucial political decision occurred in the mid-1950s, at the height of the Cold War and in a period of British decline. Previously, the synthesis of heroin in 1874 and its commer-cial marketing as a "wonder drug" had contributed to a pattern of addiction that continued into the early 1900s, with physicians, phar-macists, and patent medicine salesmen dispensing narcotics freely to patients and consumers. In 1947, the World Health Organization (WHO), under direct pressure from the United States, requested that its member countries ban the production and importation of

heroin.[*][11] By 1955, the Canadian government agreed, whereas the
British government rejected the recommendation after consultations
with the British Medical Association. During these meetings, British
physicians called heroin an "excellent sedative which is of estimable
value in so many conditions."[12] The Canadian government, for its
part, opted not to discuss the Canadian Medical Association's position during debates in the Commons. More importantly, it failed to
heed the CMA's advice. Dr A.D. Kelly, the deputy general secretary of
the CMA, provided a viewpoint supporting heroin on 23 July 1952,
which was subsequently neglected. Kelly's opinion was as follows:

> I believe that Canadian doctors feel that diacetylmorphine is a use-
> ful drug ... The Canadian profession has not been convinced that
> the elimination of heroin for medical purposes has been conspic-
> uously successful in reducing addiction, e.g. U.S.A. It is my view
> that our answer would be similar to that given two years ago.[13]

Canada's politicians ultimately chose to restrict heroin for medical
purposes in Canada, although this was not a decision taken lightly.
According to Paul Martin Sr, the federal health and welfare minister
in 1955 and father of his namesake son, the future prime minister,
"We knew heroin had its benefits. But the WHO was reporting that
it should be stopped and, since most countries were following the
recommendation, I think it made sense that we went along with it."
Still, he added, "it was definitely a frustrating decision."[14]

Kenneth Walker (aka Gifford-Jones) also found the decision
frustrating. He had lost several close friends to cancer, a number
of whom had dealt with tremendous pain. After some thought, he
came to the conclusion that much of the suffering was a product of
inadequate administration of existing analgesics as well as the unfair
restrictions on heroin. "[S]ince heroin had been used so effectively
in England, I had to ask myself why this narcotic couldn't be made
available to Canadian physicians."[15]

Walker's argument in favour of heroin was built on evidence of
the drug's effectiveness and the example of heroin's use in the UK.
It was built on a foundation of compassion and empathy for the

---

* By 1924, the US became the first country in the world to outlaw the use of heroin for
medical purposes.

victims of terminal cancer as well a broader concern for the rights
of the dying in Canada. First, heroin, he noted, was a faster-acting
analgesic compared to morphine, because it was more soluble. This
was especially important in treating patients who were so emaciated
that they had little muscle left into which to inject a drug, making
a large shot of morphine, the most widely used analgesic, extremely
painful. Second, he also argued that heroin was beneficial for those
patients troubled by the side effects of morphine, including nightmares, nausea, constipation, and hallucinations.[16]

In presenting his case to Canadians, Walker drew on the available
medical literature, much of which came from Great Britain. In doing
so, he highlighted the radically different approach to medical heroin
in the United Kingdom, which was traceable to the 1926 Rolleston
committee. That committee recommended that doctors be allowed to
prescribe narcotics to wean patients off drugs; to relieve pain after a
prolonged cure had failed; and in cases where small doses enabled
patients to perform useful tasks and lead normal lives. Britain's public
policy was modified during the 1960s, when it witnessed an upsurge
in drug addiction, resulting in the 1967 Dangerous Drug Act and
1971 Misuse of Drugs Bill, laws that represented a move towards the
American enforcement model. Be that as it may, the British government did not resort to the absolute prohibition of heroin, but allowed
for its medical use on a limited and controlled basis.*[17]

In the 1970s, a British heroin expert named Dr Robert Twycross,
who worked at St Christopher's hospice in London, authored
a series of academic papers that supported the use of heroin. He
determined that heroin was much safer in clinical practice than
previously believed, in addition to the fact that it possessed certain
practical advantages over morphine.[18] In his estimation, "[w]hen
injections are necessary diamorphine (heroin) is undoubtedly the
best and safest of all the potent narcotic analgesics and is indispens-
able in the care of a proportion of patients with advanced cancer."[19]
Using Twycross's extensive body of work, Walker pressed his case in
the popular press, with politicians, and to authorities in the medical
establishment, many of whom patently rejected his ideas.

---

* Provisions in the 1960s included: (1) addicts were forced to register with a central
authority (the Home Office); (2) disciplinary rules were introduced for doctors who
violated restrictions; (3) mandatory licensing was introduced relative to scheduled drugs.

Walker also contributed to larger debates in the realm of Canadian palliative care, specifically those about addiction, spirituality, definitions of quality of life, and specialized training.[20] Many of these issues had been pioneered by Cicely Saunders in London, England, who was a major contributor to the "evolution of the field" and whose legacy remains the growth of "the hospice movement and research into the needs of the terminally ill."[21] While drawing on her experiences in the British system, she sought to "ensure that a misplaced concern about addiction did not prevent doctors from prescribing large enough doses of opiates to relieve patients with advanced cancer."[22] Intellectually, this meant reevaluating common conceptions about spectrums of pain and medicines, including heroin. The exigencies of death required a less segmented view of end-of-life therapies and it was unhelpful to regard heroin as "the hardest drug" or as a "gentle drug."[23] In Saunders's estimation, this constituted an outmoded approach, one which Walker sought to rectify.[24]

He was also adding to a well-established record in Canadian palliative care. Between 1973 and 2004, Dr Balfour Mount, an international expert on pain in the dying, spearheaded innovative palliative care organizations and research and training at McGill University in Montreal. Following in the footsteps of Cicely Saunders in the UK, and Zelda Foster, Elisabeth Kübler-Ross, and William M. Lamers in the United States, Mount sought to provide more patient-centred holistic and humanistic care, which necessarily required a reevaluation of existing modes of care for dying patients.[25] His efforts emerged as part of a larger movement in medicine that was responding to the depersonalized care the dying received from the traditional system. He founded the International Congresses in Care of the Dying in 1976, published over fifty papers on pain in the terminally ill, has become recognized as the father of palliative care in Canada, and is often credited with coining the term "palliative care."[26] More than this, at the same university, the McGill Pain Questionnaire was developed in the 1970s by two doctors, Ronald Melzack and Warren Torgerson, and remains the main tool for measuring pain in clinics worldwide. Having already revolutionized the field of pain research in 1965 with the seminal "gate control theory," Melzack then joined forces with Torgerson and the physicians began to list the words patients used to describe their pain in the mid-1970s. They classified them into three categories:

- sensory (heat, pressure, "throbbing" or "pounding" sensations)
- affective (related to emotional effects, such as "tiring," "sickening," "gruelling," or "frightful")
- evaluative (related to experience – from "annoying and "troublesome" to "horrible," "unbearable," and "excruciating")

This work at McGill led to the most comprehensive reference book in pain medicine yet written. And it solidified the university's reputation as a global leader in the study of pain.[27]

One of the earliest opponents of heroin's legalization in Canada was the Canadian Cancer Society. The Society's National Advisory Committee had pored over the evidence and found heroin did not contain any "unique properties" and was not "needed if existing drugs are used correctly."[28] (From 1980 to 1983, Kenneth Walker and the W. Gifford-Jones Foundation paid for a series of advertisements that focused on the "dinosaur mentality" of the CCS.) The Canadian Society of Hospital Pharmacists also dismissed the therapeutic value of heroin and specifically targeted Kenneth Walker as a charlatan. The *Canadian Journal of Hospital Pharmacy*, for example, suggested that Walker was offering false hope and peddling "patent nonsense."[29] This type of argument was reiterated elsewhere. In the United States, for example, Dr Kathleen Foley chronicled how "vulnerable and desperate" cancer patients were led to believe that physicians possessed a virtual panacea. She also made the case that the excessive focus on heroin drew attention away from more vital issues, including systemic change in pain treatment regimes. Another notable opponent of heroin's legalization for medical purposes was the Royal Canadian Mounted Police, which held "that the heroin problem in Canada was extensive and on the rise." According to an RCMP report in 1984, "[w]hile the heroin user population remained stable at an estimated 20,000 users requiring approximately 175.2–255.5 kg of heroin per year, the supplier countries were re-establishing themselves, year by year, trying to increase the amount of illicit heroin supplied to Canada." In the wake of drug intelligence estimates showing a rise in the availability of heroin, the RCMP also argued against any further increase in heroin availability in Canada, something which medicinal heroin would have of course provided.[30]

LONDON CALLING: MEDICAL KNOWLEDGE
AND CANADIAN LEGISLATION

By 1982, Walker had collected 30,000 signatures on a petition calling for heroin's legalization in Canada as well as an additional 20,000 letters supporting his efforts. He had also spent a considerable amount of time conducting an investigation into the use of heroin in the UK, specifically London. During a fact-finding mission, Walker met with pain specialists, nurses, nursing sisters, and patients throughout London's hospitals, including Great Ormond Street Hospital, Royal Marsden Hospital, One Trinity Hospice, St Thomas's Hospital, and the famous St Christopher's Hospice. He also visited Scotland Yard, where officials remarked that they had much larger crime concerns than therapeutic heroin.[31] Following his tour of various hospitals and a series of interviews, Walker was further convinced that heroin was a useful tool for physicians and ought to be implemented in Canada, just as in the British health system.

At the same time, he demonstrated serious displeasure with heroin experts and pain specialists in London and elsewhere in the UK. While they were perfectly fine with sharing their medical opinions on the therapeutic value of heroin in clinical practice, Walker wrote, it was nevertheless "difficult to find a doctor willing to come to Canada and speak to my colleagues."[32] In Walker's estimation, this reluctance was a byproduct of an "old boy network" wherein invitations to Canada were rebuffed so as not to "offend" Canadian pain experts. Walker thought this contemptible, and he was scathing in his criticism, calling British doctors both dishonest and hypocritical.[33] Examples of such reluctance also occurred in the United States. The pioneering and oft-cited Dr Twycross chose not to engage in the American legislative process for the simple reason that the sanctioning of heroin in the United States would not make a marked difference. Relative to Britain, pain management and pain control in the US were limited and suffered from inadequate scheduling and limited dosing, which meant that "the doctors who use their present narcotics badly will use heroin just as badly ... patients will be no better off."[34] Heroin's legalization was a moot point in his view, since the entirety of end-of-life pain control in the American system required reform. He chose not to involve himself.

After Walker's efforts to raise awareness of heroin, in 1982 he presented his petition and letters requesting the legalization of heroin to the federal health and welfare minister, Monique Bégin, in Ottawa. This forced the government into action. Bégin duly announced the formation of the Medical Advisory Committee on the Management of Severe Pain, which was populated by physicians and academics from Canada's major research institutions. Edward Sellers, a professor of pharmacology and medicine at the University of Toronto, was named chairman, while Balfour Mount, a professor of surgery and the director of palliative care at McGill University, served as vice-chair.[35]

Walker, for his part, was skeptical. He argued that the committee members, including Mount, were largely opposed to heroin and felt it unlikely that the government would "admit it had been wrong for twenty-nine years."[36] In one of his columns, Walker suggested, "The debate [has become] a political one, not medical."[37] Also concerned that the expert committee would grind any legalization momentum to a halt, he formed the W. Gifford-Jones Foundation in early 1983 with the express purpose of galvanizing public sentiment even further in favour of heroin legalization as well as drumming up donations for advertising and promotional efforts. Walker's skepticism was partially validated in May 1983 when Minister Bégin declared that the government would initiate extended clinical trials to evaluate the efficacy of heroin relative to morphine and Dilaudid, the other commonly used cancer analgesics. Bégin stated, "Considering the enormous controversy about heroin, I thought such research was essential."[38]

Walker perceived the trials as delaying tactics and was infuriated by this. He believed there was more than enough "medical evidence already available than any other Minister could read in a lifetime."[39] Throughout 1983–84, he heightened the rhetoric in his national column, used the money donated to his foundation for full-page advertisements in major newspapers, and leaned on his friends in government. For example, Walker began to publish letters from Canadians whose loved ones had died in excruciating pain. He also ran a full-page advertisement in *The Globe and Mail* that critiqued the Canadian Cancer Society. In November 1984, the Gifford-Jones Foundation ran another ad supporting heroin's legalization, which stated boldly, "This Christmas will the real hypocrites please stand up."[40]

By this time, Walker had found various powerful allies in the press, medical establishment, and government. Newspaper editors, in particular, provided a defence of Walker. In November 1983, an editorial in *The Toronto Star* announced: "Heroin represents the most effective way some cancer patients can manage the terrible pain that can come with the disease. If these people need it, it should ... be available to them." *The Globe and Mail* also supported legalization. In June 1984, an editorial attacked the government for "30 years of delay during which cancer patients have faced the ultimate pain without heroin, which is widely used in Britain where there are no political arguments against its medicinal use."[41] The fact that both major papers supported heroin legalization suggested that this issue crossed the normally bifurcated political spectrum, *The Toronto Star* being left and *The Globe* being centre-right.

Besides the editorial boards of Canada's major newspapers, the Canadian Medical Association supported Walker's efforts. One physician, Dr William Ghent, who practised and taught at Queen's University, proved especially influential. Leading the CMA's Council on Healthcare, he exposed how deception characterized the original 1954 decision to ban heroin in Canadian medicine. In his view, Canada had succumbed to American pressures and government ministers, including Paul Martin Sr, had misled colleagues by suggesting that the CMA supported prohibition.[42] In August 1984, the CMA's general council recommended that physicians be authorized to prescribe heroin, the time being right for Canada to join the thirty-six other countries using heroin in a medical fashion. "Heroin was banned," Ghent argued, "on the naïve assumption by government and its police forces that if all heroin was illegal, prosecution would be easier and thus illicit use of the drug would be eradicated."[43] Much more vividly, he added: "We followed the U.S. like sheep and now, like sheep, we've got their manure to deal with."[44]

The Liberal government's expert committee agreed with neither Ghent nor the CMA – quite the opposite, in fact. In September 1984, the Medical Advisory Committee on the Management of Severe Pain released its report and recommended that heroin "not be reintroduced at this time since the information available does not support the need for this drug."[45] Instead, the committee argued that the primary barrier to pain control was not a lack of effective analgesics but the fact that most doctors and nurses were poorly trained in pain control. The committee also argued that physicians and nurses, because of their belief in and reliance on drugs, neglected to use alternative methods of pain control and failed to assess patients' emotional and mental conditions.[46] In short, the fundamental causes behind inadequate pain control would not be addressed by heroin;

thus, the panel placed an emphasis on better understanding and improvement of accepted painkillers such as Dilaudid. Dr Gifford-Jones called the panel "biased" in the national press.[47]

Of course, much of this report was lost in the wake of the landmark Canadian election, which was held on 4 September. The Liberal Party's long-standing dominance was severely eroded under the leadership of John Turner. It would remain to be seen how Brian Mulroney's new Conservative government, now holding a formidable 282 seats in Parliament, would treat the issue of medical heroin. Yet, for Walker there were reasons to hope. First, Jake Epp, the new health and welfare minister, was familiar with the debates, having served on a standing committee which examined the need for heroin in hospitals and was apparently sympathetic to the measure. Second, the committee itself was formed after Conservative MP James McGrath introduced an underreported, dead-on-arrival bill to decriminalize heroin for medical use in April 1983. While this bill had gone nowhere in a Liberal-controlled Parliament, throughout the fall he developed a close relationship with Epp over the issue.[48] They discussed the RCMP's opposition to the measure and the expert committee's report, in addition to questioning the need for the further clinical trials that Minister Bégin had initiated.

Then, a month after the federal election in October 1984, the Ontario legislature unanimously passed a motion that urged the new Conservative federal government to legalize heroin. The issues on which many of the Ontario assembly touched included Great Britain's use of heroin, unfounded fears that it would seep onto Canadian streets, and worries about addiction. Vincent Kerrio, a Liberal MPP and friend and ally of Kenneth Walker, had put forward the motion and led discussions. In his introductory remarks, he referenced British experiences of medical heroin:

> We know that English doctors have been using heroin for more than 80 years. This is the best trial that has ever been done. Why do we not believe them and put an end to these committees and costly studies? Consider, for instance, that in 1982 English doctors used 98.7 per cent of the legal heroin consumed in the entire world, not forgetting that these doctors had a choice of painkillers.[49]

Kerrio's colleague from St Catharines, Mr Bradley, also added that the British example was valuable to acknowledge when considering therapeutic heroin. "The British use it," he noted. And "the British are not foolish people in the treatment of their patients." He then addressed concerns about addiction:

> Many have mentioned the problem of addiction and many have stated in this House today how foolish it is to worry about addiction to the use of heroin of those who are in their last days before death and are in greatest pain. Frankly, who cares if they are addicted to heroin at that time?[50]

CANADIAN HEROIN POLICY

Jake Epp consulted with his fellow Conservatives throughout the fall and maintained a strong working relationship with McGrath. To that point, heroin had proven an intriguing area of debate within the healthcare sector, as well as with law enforcement and the public. The RCMP was against the limited and controlled legalization of the drug, as were other organizations, including the Canadian Cancer Society and the Canadian Society of Hospital Pharmacists. The medical establishment largely supported the move, as did a significant number of Canadian citizens.

Epp found himself in a position in which he had to choose between the Canadian Medical Association's recommendation and that made by the former government's expert advisory committee. "It is not a technical question which we are addressing," he stated, "but rather the meaning of life and how death with dignity can be enhanced."[51] The decision, in these terms, was straightforward. On 20 December, he announced that the government would legalize the use of heroin in cases of severe chronic pain or terminal illness. Afterward, Epp declared he was not convinced legal heroin posed a threat to the safety of Canadians or that substance abuse would increase. He had challenged "law enforcement agencies to show me one case anywhere in the world where street addiction had gone up because heroin was legally available in hospitals."[52] Apparently, an example could not be found. For McGrath, he suggested that the Liberal government's expert advisory committee, led by Edward Sellers and Balfour Mount, was "biased" and "stacked with known opponents of heroin." "It was like Chrysler or Ford looking into Japanese cars."[53]

Yet, the committee's views on heroin were not simple nor simply a product of bias. Balfour Mount worked tirelessly throughout his long and influential career to promote more progressive and complex approaches to pain treatment. After training with Cicely Saunders in London, he began to view pain treatment as an interaction of physical, psychological, social, and spiritual elements. One drug, whether heroin or morphine, was not sufficient to approach this complicated experience. His resistance to heroin, in short, was based on a philosophy of palliative care and pain management that was about more than just drugs. Heroin, in his view, distracted from more crucial issues in palliative care. The fight over the drug's legitimacy meant that less attention was given to anticipating pain. The struggle about heroin, in short, was about the very final stages of life, when *all* of the stages ought to be accounted for in a critical way. According to Mount, "Waiting for pain to reappear before treating it only perpetuates the fear of pain and the need for higher analgesic doses. It's a vicious cycle."[54] Heroin, for him, was part of a cycle that he hoped to break.

Kenneth Walker, as one might imagine, celebrated the Conservative government's decision. In advocating for the legalization of heroin at the end of life, he had criticized the medical community for its failure to rethink its myths and prejudices about drugs and suffering terminal cancer patients. His effort to make heroin available was a partial solution and he did not claim, as many accused him of doing, that it would solve all the problems associated with terminal cancer pain. Walker insisted that the patient's pain be situated at the centre of care and the patient's choices be increased. He also underlined how an unjustified panic about narcotics for those same patients was accompanied by narrow-mindedness in the medical establishment.[55] Overall, he asked valuable questions about the experience and nature of suffering and challenged others to ruminate on how cancer patients conducted themselves in the face of pain. Even more, he challenged medical professionals to engage with the patients' pain.

In a broader sense, Canada's legalization of heroin represented a return of colonial medicine. Canadian medical authorities and politicians continually referenced the British use of heroin for chronic pain or in end-of-life situations, using both medical literature and the more subjective patient and physician testimonials. To be sure, the therapeutic use of heroin in the UK was what initially prompted Kenneth Walker to begin his quest for legalization and, following this, he founded much of his argument on Britain's heroin history. This was a comeback for colonial medicine, as Canadians began to take cues from the mother country, whether it was through Saunders, Twycross, or the BMA's rejection of the heroin ban in the 1950s. Even the rejection of heroin by the expert advisory committee signalled a renaissance in British influence on Canadian medical practice as well as progress on the understanding of the drug. Balfour Mount, one of the world's foremost thinkers on palliative care treatment, trained in London with Saunders and viewed proper end-of-life and pain treatments as far more complex than a simple panacea.

Consequently, as US politicians, medical authorities, and health activists debated and then ultimately rejected heroin as a part of legitimate hospice care, Canadians adopted it. While Americans used rhetoric about heroin infiltrating the streets and legislative efforts were overwhelmingly defeated, in Canada heroin was made available. The influence of the UK proved too powerful. The newly elected Conservative government chose a radically different approach from Republican policy-makers in the US.

As the relatively recent case in British Columbia over heroin-assisted therapy illustrates, however, the contestation over heroin in medical circles and in society more generally has not ended. Some citizens were scandalized by the prospect of heroin therapy for addicts. Others were fine with the prospect of administering heroin. Health authorities and policy-makers must grapple with the con-troversial therapy, which is designed for addiction maintenance and crime-prevention purposes. Studies produced by the North American Opiate Medication Initiative (NAOMI) fifteen years ago offered mainly positive results for severe addicts who have resisted tradi-tional methadone treatments. Yet, there has been little policy move-ment in this direction, meaning the contest over heroin therapy in Canada will likely continue in the years ahead. As this occurs, it may be useful to once again draw on the British experience. John Marks, for example, a physician in Wales during Margaret Thatcher's anti-drug campaigns in the 1980s who initiated a research program that provided heroin to four hundred addicts, produced some startling outcomes. His experiment with heroin-assisted therapy was meant to demonstrate that his clinic possessed a cost-effective anti-drug strategy, but it ultimately showed that there were no heroin-related deaths and theft and burglary dropped by 93 percent.[56] While his experiment was ignored and he was blacklisted in Britain, Canadian health authorities have the opportunity to once again take lessons on medical heroin from the mother country.

JUSTIFYING JUNK: HEROIN IN THE AMERICAN HOSPICE DURING REAGAN'S WAR ON DRUGS

"I have learned the junk equation," wrote William S. Burroughs in his semi-autobiographical 1953 book, *Junkie*. "Junk is not, like alcohol or weed, a means to increase enjoyment of life. Junk is not a kick. It is a way of life." According to Burroughs, the beatnik, spoken word performer, and author of other books such as *Naked Lunch* and *Queer*, heroin was not simply a drug that enhanced the quality of one's everyday experiences. Nor was it a means to be a more productive individual.[1] By the end of the 1970s as well as throughout the 1980s, the discussion over heroin moved beyond the exclusive realm of recreational use (and misuse) by Punks, New Yorkers, Vietnam veterans, and Burroughs's narrow conception. Amid the "war on cancer" and "war on drugs," an eclectic mix of activists, physicians, and politicians in the US and Canada argued that heroin ought to constitute part of the pain management regime for individuals afflicted with terminal cancer. With the publication of studies that found heroin superior to morphine and the British health system's implementation of heroin treatment in the 1970s, medical, law enforcement, and political authorities came into conflict with interest groups. According to its advocates, heroin was a humane solution for terminally ill cancer patients suffering through tremendous amounts of pain. Junk, in this instance, was therapy, not a "kick." It was a tool to manage death in a respectful and appropriate way, rather than a way of life. More broadly, the struggle embodied long-standing debates about patient-consumer choice in the medical marketplace, heroin as a valid analgesic, and conceptions of pain in the United States, as well as the racial meanings of heroin. According to Judith Quattlebaum, the founder of the largest health activist organization driving the legalization effort, the Committee for the Treatment for Intractable Pain (CTIP), "It is time we Americans give up our excessive fear of heroin ... Its legitimate use, when death is close, outweighs its total prohibition on grounds of abuse in any thoughtful ethical formulation."[2]

Heroin, which of course has a distinct history in the United States relative to Canada, helps us to understand culture, ideology, and the politics of pain management during the 1970s and 1980s. For historian Keith Wailoo, conservatives during the Reagan era employed the rhetoric of "learned helplessness" and attacked disability aid. In his estimation, "there was in fact such thing as a *liberal pain standard* that had been developed within disability policy, in medicine and science, and in government during the decades before Reagan became president, and there was, in his own time, a severe backlash aiming to impose a *conservative standard* for judging pain."[3] Heroin highlighted stark ideological divisions at the bedside, in Congress, and in the scientific community, and it also complicates Wailoo's view of a bifurcated politics of pain.

Just as important, overlapping with this was the rise of the hospice movement, which had its genesis in the mid-1960s. It was bound up in and bolstered by the larger social, economic, and political changes of the period and sought to answer questions about the appropriate treatment of dying Canadians and Americans. This was an era in which the dying were accorded more rights, and changing attitudes towards the dying duly influenced conceptions of heroin. Zelda Foster, Elisabeth Kübler-Ross, and other North American medical practitioners advocated for reform of orthodox end-of-life care, asking questions about the experience and nature of suffering and challenging others to ruminate on how cancer patients conducted themselves in the face of pain.

Contrary to conventional wisdom, the political reaction to heroin was far more convoluted than one might assume; it was qualified and sustained by scientific delierations, if not rock-solid judgments. As Democratic and Republican lawmakers in the United States sponsored legislation providing irrevocably sick individuals in hospices limited access to heroin, physicians and clinical researchers rigorously debated the science behind and ethics of administering heroin to palliative care patients in the pages of *The Lancet*, the *New England Journal of Medicine*, and the *Annals of Internal Medicine*. Ultimately, heroin treatment obtained support from many conservative Republicans, which in turn complicates orthodox views of the War on Drugs and

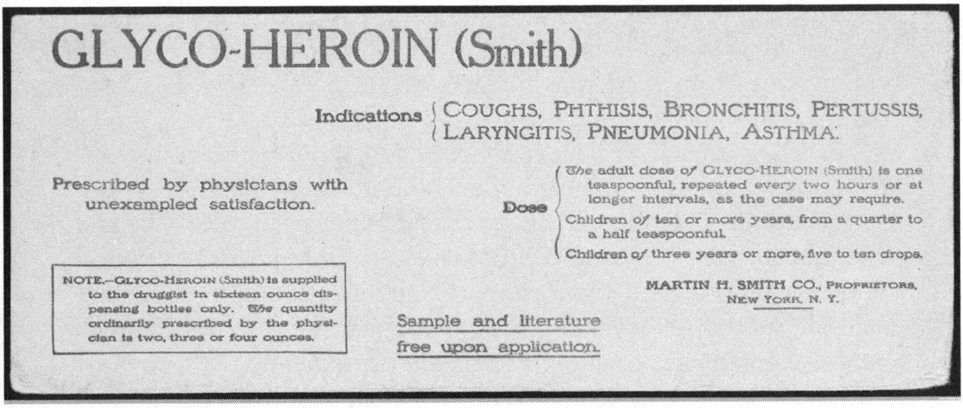

GLYCO-HEROIN (Smith)

Indications { COUGHS, PHTHISIS, BRONCHITIS, PERTUSSIS,
LARYNGITIS, PNEUMONIA, ASTHMA.

Prescribed by physicians with
unexampled satisfaction.

Dose {
The adult dose of GLYCO-HEROIN (Smith) is one
teaspoonful, repeated every two hours or at
longer intervals, as the case may require.
Children of ten or more years, from a quarter to
a half teaspoonful.
Children of three years or more, five to ten drops.

NOTE.—GLYCO-HEROIN (Smith) is supplied
to the druggist in sixteen ounce dispensing bottles only. The quantity
ordinarily prescribed by the physician is two, three or four ounces.

MARTIN H. SMITH CO., PROPRIETORS.
NEW YORK, N. Y.

Sample and literature
free upon application.

FIGURE 2.1 Heroin advertisement. Used for various indications, including bronchitis, coughs, pertussis, and others, heroin was synthesized in 1874. Wellcome Trust Images, Martin H. Smith Co., New York., circa 1900s.

modern American conservatism more broadly. For example, William F. Buckley Jr, a founding father of the American conservative revival after the Second World War and surely among its leading intellectual figures, championed the use of heroin for the terminally ill. He was not the only high-profile conservative of the era to suggest that the law ought to be modified. Breaking from the standard anti-drug orthodoxy, such US senators as Robert Dole, Barry Goldwater, Orrin Hatch, and Ernest Hollings, among others, promoted the use of heroin by legitimate palliative specialists to assist with cancer pain.

In contrast, certain liberal Democrats, including Representative Charles Rangel (D-NY), maintained strict opposition to heroin's use for cancer pain. His opposition was driven by concern for African-American drug users in his native Harlem, a matter that had occupied him since 1971, when he first won the district. Addiction and its solution, including methadone use, had developed as a policy issue for black political leaders during Vietnam and rightfully carried over into the 1980s. In short, the category of race was obvious in the discussion of heroin legislation.[4] According to legal scholar Kenneth Nunn, it is possible to view anti-drug strategies through the prism of ethnicity. During the War on Drugs, "race played an important role over the years in identifying the communities that became the targets of the drug war, consequently exposing their cultural practices and institutions to military-style attack and police control."[5]

Curiously, during the debate over heroin as a cancer treatment, African-American political leaders were the individuals "identifying communities," an issue that further challenges and revamps standard views of the War on Drugs.

In a larger sense, any historical discussion about heroin as a treatment for terminally ill cancer patients should be located within two so-called "wars" (on drugs and cancer) that began in the 1960s and continue into the present. Within this setting and under these conditions, heroin occupied a unique space in political, cultural, and medical spheres, where it was regarded as "the hardest drug" of them all as well as a "gentle drug" in possession of tremendous therapeutic potential. Heroin was simultaneously a social problem *and* solution, a scourge *and* saviour.[6]

NIXON'S WARS: DRUG CAREERS AND CANCER

The synthesis of heroin in 1874 and its commercial marketing as a "wonder drug" contributed to a pattern of addiction that continued into the early 1900s, with physicians, pharmacists, and patent medicine salesmen dispensing narcotics freely to patients and consumers. This simple chemical compound had been restricted to legitimate medical use only by the Harrison Narcotic Act of 1914. Then, in 1924, prodded by public and professional hysteria, Congress passed a law that prohibited the importation of opium for the purpose of manufacturing heroin. The intent was to outlaw heroin, and, in fact, the legitimate use of the drug diminished greatly. Despite widespread beliefs to the contrary, however, heroin remained legal in American medicine until 18 November 1956, when it was totally outlawed.[7]

When illegal recreational drugs such as heroin intersect with the mainstream medical marketplace, drug users and regulators, oncologists and palliative care specialists, as well as researchers, law enforcement officials, and the public, must negotiate the conditions under which evidence shapes policy. For Arnold Trebach, all of the arguments in favour of heroin's prohibition in the US were moral, political, ideological, and criminological, rather than scientific.*[8]

---

* Still, science can be easily mediated by outside forces. According to *Buzzed*, most interpretations of the scientific literature relevant to drugs such as heroin are "oversimplified, inaccurate, or disseminated by organizations that slant the research to further political and moral agendas."

According to Carnwath and White, the dispute over heroin in the 1980s aroused such passion because it linked cancer, the most feared disease, with heroin, the most feared drug of the era.[9] Yet, at the outset of the 1970s, Richard M. Nixon was bellicose in the face of such implacable foes. While he was already prosecuting a war in Southeast Asia, Nixon declared that he – and the United States – would stand firm against threats to Americans' health. Neither cancer nor drugs (including the dreaded heroin) would conquer America, and he announced a "war" on both.[10] During his 1971 State of the Union Address, Nixon boldly pronounced, much like John F. Kennedy had with space travel to the moon, that Americans would lead the way. Nixon suggested his nation's medical establishment, supported by the government, would "launch an intensive campaign to fund a cure for cancer." Thereafter, Nixon signed into law the National Cancer Act, which broadened the scope and responsibilities of the National Cancer Institute, and expanded federal funding "in order to more effectively carry out the national effort against cancer."[11] Since then, over 100 billion dollars of federal research grants have been consumed by this effort, and yet the "War on Cancer" has been declared a failure, in both medical literature and news coverage.

In contrast to the marked success of cholesterol-lowering drugs and antihypertensives in reducing the risk of cardiovascular disease, Daniel Haber et al. write, the decline in cancer mortality has been relatively modest.* According to *Nature Medicine*, "with few exceptions, treatments haven't lived up to expectations."[12] When President Richard Nixon first declared a war on cancer in 1971, there were high hopes not only that scientists stood on the threshold of understanding the underlying causes of cancer, but that many cures were within reach. This, of course, did not prove to be the case. What has changed in recent times is the cancer metaphor. Until recently, the metaphor has been that of an invading army, a barbarian horde attacking from outside the city walls.[13]

In the 1950s, medical researchers saw cancer as "an extremely complicated process that needed to be described in hundreds, if not thousands of different ways," Weinberg says. "The war on cancer

---

* This decrease has been attributed primarily to screening for breast and colon cancer and preventive measures, such as a reduction in smoking and the declining use of post-menopausal estrogen replacement.

will not be won in one dramatic battle, it will be a series of skir-mishes." In current parlance, the war on cancer would not be won by full-scale combat, but rather would be asymmetric warfare won by small, incremental victories. Scientists started glimpsing what they thought were simplifying principles. The first idea, which helped spur the government's war on cancer, was that viruses were the prime drivers of human cancers. That proved not to be the case. "Over the last 10 to 15 years we began to accumulate once again an over-whelming mass of information that cancer is indeed a highly com-plex process, and that attempts at distilling it down to a small num-ber of simple processes may not really work that easily," Weinberg says. "And so we're once again caught in this quandary: How can we understand this complexity in terms of a small number of underly-ing basic principles?"[14] At the inaugural International Evolution and Cancer Conference in 2011, several researchers, including Steven Neuberg, proposed a new way of thinking about the disease. He likened cancer cells to local residents who have gone bad and then slowly exploit the environment around them for their own gain. Accordingly, instead of external forces or "foreign invaders," "crim-inal gangs" was a more apt metaphor for cancer. "Cancers are not outside the body," Neuberg says. "They come from within us."[15]

Similarly, the Nixon administration interpreted drug addiction and the heroin scourge as a product of *both* foreign invaders and criminal gangs, from Turkey and Mexico to Harlem and the Bronx. Meanwhile, public awareness of heroin grew in American society for a number of reasons. There were celebrity deaths (Janis Joplin, 1970, and Jim Morrison, 1971). Major motion pictures (*Jennifer on My Mind*, 1971; *Midnight Cowboy*, 1969; *More*, 1969; *The French Connection*, 1971; *The Panic in Needle Park*, 1971) focused on heroin. What's more, the publication of congressional reports high-lighted that American GIs were addicted to high-grade heroin. As far-flung as these political and cultural events were, they intersected and gave force to anti-heroin sentiment. The government launched a "big and bold" drug war, which, according to *Science*, was "basi-cally a war on heroin."[16] And popular culture, in short, reinterpreted, translated, and ultimately galvanized ideas about heroin's dangers in the late 1960s and early 1970s.

Such was the reality that following the Comprehensive Drug Abuse and Prevention Control Act of 1970's passage, in June of 1971, Nixon officially declared a War on Drugs and called drug abuse "enemy number one in America."[17] That same year, Nixon created the Special Action Office for Drug Abuse Prevention (SAODAP) within the Executive Office of the President as a "dramatic way to highlight the problem." In 1973, the National Institute of Drug Abuse was established. During this period, the national treatment effort jumped from $18 to 350 million between 1966 and 1975, while methadone morphed from an experimental opioid to a legitimate treatment method. In the short term, President Nixon's initiatives produced results. An East Coast heroin shortage in 1973, mixed with dwindling lines of heroin addicts seeking treatment, signalled a victory of sorts. Quick to claim victory, Nixon declared that a "corner had been turned." This was inaccurate, and certain inner-city areas within New York, Boston, and Washington, DC, began to suffer alarmingly high overdose rates in 1974. With federal funding levelling off, by as early as 1974 the problem of heroin (emerging from Mexico) was "coming back in full force."[18] According to social scientist James Q. Wilson, the "crisis mentality" that was associated with heroin in the early 1970s, like any other strong passion, could not endure. Heroin seemed localized to ghetto areas and when the problem touched the "lives of comparatively few people," the public, press, and national politicians let the matter "slip away." For Wilson, "the popular mind deals with the heroin problem as it deals with horror movies – alternately fascinated and repelled, but ultimately bored, and so its attention is episodic."[19]

PAIN, HEROIN, AND HOSPICE HISTORY

The American hospice movement, which had its genesis in the mid-1960s, was bolstered by the larger socio-economic and political trends of the period. It sought to answer questions about the appropriate treatment of dying Americans and pushed back against fear of the reaper, *non timetis messor*. Yet, the humane treatment and alternative approach to pain relief that was embodied in the movement found a barrier in the politicization of pain in the 1980s. This was an era of widespread political activist movements focused on the Vietnam War, civil rights for blacks, the plight of American Indians, and feminism; together these groups reinforced and propelled health activism.[20] Within this milieu, numerous advocates, including Kübler-Ross and others mentioned above, pushed to change the status quo. Part of the effort was to identify with the patient's experience, to place them at the centre of the end-of-life treatment model. Even more, advocates asked medical professionals to engage with the patients' pain, and to ponder whether it was necessary to immerse themselves in suffering or adopt a cold professional detachment.

The earliest impetus for hospice programming in the US can be traced to the famous British physician and spokeswoman, Cicely Saunders, who in the early 1960s embarked on "an exhausting schedule of speaking and teaching engagements" which saw her encourage the development of new hospice programs.[21] Following her instrumental tour in the late 1960s and early 1970s, the hospice movement slowly gained momentum "in an unsystematic and largely unplanned manner" throughout the decade, and by the mid-1980s the number of hospices had ballooned to roughly 1,500.[22] A "diversity of organizational structure" typified these hospices and three organizational models emerged: the freestanding hospice model, the home health agency-based model, and the hospital-based model.[23] The definition of "hospice," as cited by the American National Hospice Organization, is "a medically directed multidisciplinary program providing skilled care of an appropriate nature for terminally ill patients and their families to live as fully as possible until the time of death." As well, the hospice "helps relieve symptoms during the distress (physical, psychological, spiritual, social, economic) that may occur during the course of the disease, dying, and bereavement."[24]

Ultimately, the tremendous growth and reification of the movement would not have been possible without key intellectual forces at such institutions as Yale University, for example, or through its tireless championing by Florence Wald, William M. Lamers, and numerous others. Zelda Foster, a native New Yorker, a product of Columbia University, and supervisor of social work at Veterans Administration Medical Center in Brooklyn, authored an influential paper in 1965 that critiqued what she called the "conspiracy of silence" facing dying patients in hospitals.[25] No longer able to ignore the poor treatment of the terminally ill, she pressed hospital staff to address the psychological needs of patients, meaning a focus on the lack of information provided to them, their isolation from family members, and their silent submission to their fate. It was a call for empowering the dying patient.[26]

Even more famous was Elisabeth Kübler-Ross, who produced the bestselling *On Death and Dying* in 1969. According to the *British*

Medical Journal, the book "rocked the medical profession and at the same time also resulted in a public outcry for compassionate care of the dying." Just like Foster, Kübler-Ross emphasized communication; through dialogue, patients could review "their lives, their deterioration, and imminent death ... a good death could be achieved."[27] Moreover, Kübler-Ross promoted the five-stage framework of death and dying, which comprised denial, anger, bargaining, depression, and acceptance, and she pressed the medical community to employ it.[28]

In broad terms, the hospice, according to Paradis and Cummings, was originally designed as a refuge or a "way station" for terminally ill patients and their families. Not only was it to provide more patient-centred holistic and humanistic care, but the goals of the hospice required a reevaluation of existing modes of care for dying patients.[29] The hospice movement in the United States emerged as a reaction to the depersonalized care the dying received from the traditional medical system, which often failed to relieve the pain and discomfort associated with cancer and cancer-related treatment. "Pain," as described by Keith Wailoo, "came to represent not just a clinical or scientific problem, but a legal puzzle, a heated cultural concern, and an enduring partisan issue."[30]

By the mid-1980s (when heroin treatments and legislation were being discussed), the larger hospice movement and hospice founders challenged technological interventionism, the lack of communication among care-givers and patients, and the needless prolonging of life. Hospices, in short, were about patient and family choice and were viewed as a "constructive alternative to the patient ... when further aggressive therapy could not promise hope of remission or cure."[31] At the same time, the hospice movement was also perceived as a "vehicle through which selected aspects of the American medical system could be transformed."[32] More specifically, Cicely Saunders and Dr Robert Twycross also helped reformulate ideas about addiction. Saunders, drawing on her experiences in the British system, sought to "ensure that a misplaced concern about addiction did not prevent doctors from prescribing large enough doses of opiates to relieve patients with advanced cancer."[33] Intellectually, this meant reevaluating common conceptions about spectrums of pain and medicines, including heroin. The exigencies of death required a less segmented view of end-of-life therapies and it was unhelpful to regard heroin as "the hardest drug" or as a "gentle drug."[34] In Saunders's estimation, this constituted an outmoded approach.

HEROIN FOR THE DYING:
ADVOCACY AND RESISTANCE

In the wake of heroin's resurgence in 1974 and the steady growth of
the hospice movement, Judith Quattlebaum established the Committee on the Treatment of Intractable Pain (CTIP), exactly one hundred
years after the drug had first been synthesized. A life-long Republican,
Quattlebaum, at an early age, had witnessed the agonizing death of
her grandmother from cancer and decided to advocate on behalf of
a more humane and patient-centred model for dying patients. The
experience had clearly resonated with her, as she later recounted her
grandmother's cries for relief. At the peak of its strength, the lobby
organization, which was run out of Quattlebaum's home in Bethesda,
MD, had a membership of 6,000 and found support in both the Democratic and Republican parties. In particular, Quattlebaum believed
that physicians should have the right to use heroin to lessen the
dreadful pain that accompanies terminal cancer, and she often used
her supporters' letters as inspiration. "My husband," one correspon-
dent told Quattlebaum, "has been in constant pain with cancer of the
lung, which has spread to the bones, the spinal column and the brain.
Perhaps some of the people who are opposed to giving heroin should
have to watch a person suffering day after day."[35] Girded by such
pleas, Quattlebaum worked to shape conceptions about the experience of the terminal patient. "Pain," she wrote, was "soul destroy-
ing. No patient should have to endure intense pain unnecessarily."
She added, "Where doctors have a choice, both patients and doctors
prefer heroin."[36] While this rhetoric was certainly typical of a lobby
group, it was accurate in that systemic problems in the American medical establishment hindered the interpretations and treatments of pain.
According to Judy Foreman, the US medical system has done a "terrible job" of educating doctors about pain.[37]

Quattlebaum's support for of heroin was built on evidence of the
drug's effectiveness, heroin's use in the UK, and a bedrock of compassion and empathy for the victims of terminal cancer. She noted
that heroin was a faster-acting analgesic compared to morphine,
because it was more soluble. "You can use half a cc of heroin, when
you may have to use 20 times as much morphine," she told *Time*
magazine. Dosage was especially important in treating thin patients
who had little muscle left into which to inject a drug. Heroin, she
also argued, was beneficial for those patients troubled by the side

effects of morphine, including nightmares, nausea, constipation, and hallucinations.[38]

Neither a scientist nor a physician, Quattlebaum nonetheless drew on the available medical literature, much of which came from Great Britain. And she found support among her fellow Republicans, both inside and outside of Congress. One of her most articulate and influential champions was William F. Buckley Jr, the founder of *National Review*, a syndicated columnist in the US and one of the country's leading conservative intellectuals. Between 1978 and 1988, and then after her death in 2006, Buckley offered a defence of heroin in the hospice as well as praise for Quattlebaum's plucky efforts. In describing the struggle for legalization, he colourfully noted the need for meaningful policy change:

> up against the conventional unbudgability of the law which, with that magisterial irrelevance of which it is so regularly capable, in effect authorizes the use of heroin only for teenagers in ghettoes who have relatively little trouble acquiring it – while their grandmothers die in pain under the hygienic auspices of the law.[39]

Over the course of the 1970s and early 1980s, he established himself as an open-minded, unconventional conservative, and his support of the CTIP aligned with his broader avant-garde views on drug policy in the United States. With regard to drugs, he leaned on his fiscal conservatism and criticized Republicans' unwillingness to address illegal substances – the War on Drugs – through the lens of economics. As he put it in a letter in 1985, "the only logical action, unless we wish to give the Mafia, Raul Castro, and the Mexican graftocrats an unlimited lease on life, is to let the poisons fall to their natural price in an unobstructed market."[40] This meant, of course, legalization, which in turn required jettisoning moral conservatism. Often, he had little patience for such moralizing. In "Drugs, Drugs Everywhere – And No Solution in Sight," written in 1985, he repeated his proposal to legalize drugs as an alternative to unsuccessful punitive enforcement measures, yet in doing so was critical of his readers.[41] He had received countless letters elucidating the horrors of drug addiction and was exhausted by the intransigence as well as the intellectual laziness of his audience – "as though I had been arguing in favor of addiction." Drug use and addiction presented a troubling problem to policy-makers, but, he concluded, "it is not a part of any solution to write me a letter to tell me how awful drugs are."[42] He felt the same about lawmakers in Washington. Buckley often pointed out a general unwillingness to move beyond simple biases and faulty logic involved in assessing drug policy. In doing this, he, like Quattlebaum, was concerned in transcending the myths, half-truths, and fear surrounding various drugs.

Several attempts to pass a heroin bill were defeated during the 1980s. In 1984, H.R. 4762 Compassionate Pain Relief Act, sponsored by Henry Waxman (D-CA) in the House of Representatives, was approved at the committee level, whereas a companion bill in the Senate was proposed by Orrin Hatch (R-UT) and quickly found the support of diverse political leaders, including Barry Goldwater (R-AZ) and Bob Dole (R-KS). Waxman was an established proponent of consumer safety and was considered to be one of the more liberal members of the House; on various occasions, he had taken firm stances on the pharmaceutical industry and insisted that "we must assure that every drug is safe and effective" as "[t]he public expects and deserves nothing less."[43]

By this time, Waxman and Senator Orrin Hatch had formed a peculiar and formidable political relationship. In 1981, during a House-Senate conference on orphan drug legislation, they "discovered that if they worked together, they could do almost anything." Of course the two legislators were vastly different individuals: Waxman was short, bald, and moustachioed; moreover, he was a Democrat who possessed a 95 percent voter rating, according to the liberal Americans for Democratic Action. Hatch, by contrast, was tall, lean, a Mormon bishop, and a Republican whose voting record had a 95 percent rating from the conservative Americans for Constitutional Action. Their political relationship was so anomalous, so weirdly absurd, that after the passage of their significant pharmaceutical bill, the 1984 Drug Price Competition and Patent Restoration Act, generic drug manufacturers jokingly presented them with nightshirts reading "Politics Makes Strange Bedfellows."[44] For all their differences, Waxman and Hatch held shared beliefs about finding a reasonable drug policy. Both men agreed that their concerns about "health" trumped their deep "political and philosophical differences." According to Hatch, "Henry and I expect to establish a health policy that will satisfy both liberals and conservatives."[45]

The bill was designed to authorize the use of heroin over a four-year evaluation period for hospitalized terminally ill cancer patients. It was a piece of legislation directed at research and answering long-standing questions about the viability of heroin, although to critics it still represented a contravention of the 1961 Single Convention on Narcotic Drugs and a World Health Organization Agreement aimed at discontinuing the medical use of heroin due to the drug's addiction-producing qualities. For William Beaver, a pharmacologist at Georgetown in 1984, the four-year trial period was sensible – and the exigencies of scientific medicine seemed to trump other considerations. "We don't know if one patient in 10,000 will benefit (from heroin), but we ought to find out." In underlining "The Value in Heroin," the *New York Times* also endorsed the bill in its editorial section.[46] Seemingly, Quattlebaum would soon see her mission fulfilled.

It would not be for a lack of effort. She consistently contacted members of the Senate in order to lobby political support on behalf of Hatch's bill, which was designed to relieve "discomfort and pain by the therapeutic use of heroin under carefully controlled circumstances."[47] In a letter to Senator Bob Dole, the future senate leader and presidential candidate, Quattlebaum underlined support for CTIP in Kansas and urged Dole to co-sponsor the bill.[48] For his part, Dole would agree to co-sponsor Hatch's bill, putting his name down alongside other notable Republicans. The bill, however, faced robust opposition. The American Medical Association, the American Hospital Association, and the Reagan administration, along with various medical experts, expressed serious reservations about the passage of the legislation. One part of their recalcitrance toward the bill rested on skepticism of heroin's effectiveness, which had served as a point of dispute in the medical community, while another part was based on the multiple social, political, and racial meanings of heroin. The question of whether terminally ill patients would benefit from the availability of heroin was subsumed by fears that medicinal heroin would find its way onto the streets of New York and other cities.

Heroin's efficacy in mitigating pain had remained a matter of dispute since the late 1970s. In the pages of the *Annals of Internal Medicine*, the *British Journal of Addiction*, *The Lancet*, the *Journal of Contemporary Health Law & Policy*, and the *New England Journal of Medicine*, researchers and physicians debated the findings of Dr Twycross. Along with other researchers, he posited that heroin use by cancer patients did not lead to the impairment of mental functions, tolerance was not a practical problem, psychological dependence did not occur, and physical dependence was possible.

But, on this last point, dependence did not appear to prevent "the downward adjustment of the dose of heroin when considered clinically feasible."[49] Other studies demonstrated the greater lipid solubility of heroin, which led to rapid absorption into the bloodstream and an easier passage through the blood-brain barrier.[50]

By 1980, homegrown studies, sanctioned by the government, began to emerge. To considerable fanfare, a 1981 Georgetown Medical Center scientific trial had cancer patients rate morphine and heroin in easing their pain and it was revealed they rated heroin as 2.5 times more potent. The patients, moreover, did not experience euphoria. As *Science News* reported, "heroin appears to be no more addictive to cancer patients than is morphine and considerably more effective in relieving pain."[51] The team at Georgetown also discovered that heroin, having greater potency and solubility, would be useful in treating patients who had developed a high tolerance to other drugs. In 1982, a study from Memorial Sloan-Kettering Cancer Center in New York City added to the findings from Georgetown. The investigators reported that heroin was nearly twice as potent as morphine; it provided an analgesic effect earlier; doses with equal analgesic effects provided comparable improvements in moods; peak mood improvement occurred earlier after administration of heroin; and both analgesic and mood improvement were less sustained after heroin administration. Most damningly, the study held that heroin did not possess any unique advantages or disadvantages for the relief of pain.[52] Robert F. Kaiko, a pharmacologist, told *Science*, "There is no reason to believe that heroin is any more effective than morphine or that heroin is capable of relieving pain to a greater degree than is morphine." If anything, the drugs were comparable. Thereafter, in aping the language and turns of phrase from CTIP, he twisted the message of pro-heroin supporters. "There's mythology surrounding drugs," but "I hate to see people have the impression that heroin is unique. It is not unique and should be treated so."[53] Kaiko presented himself as the myth-buster. Adding further weight to this position was a colleague of Kaiko's, Kathleen Foley, chief of pain service at Memorial Sloan-Kettering, who added: the "evidence would suggest that heroin is the great non-issue of our day."[54] Similarly, according to Louis Lasagna, in his article for the *New England Journal of Medicine*, "Heroin: A Medical Me-Too," "a difference has to be enough of a difference to be a difference."[55]

What was lost in this less favourable study and its attending press coverage was that comparability did not necessarily detract from

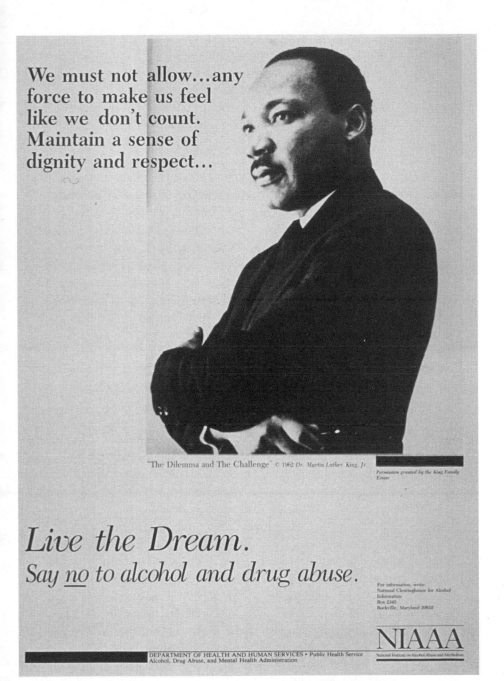

FIGURE 2.2 "Live the Dream: Say no to alcohol and drug abuse."
Rockville, MD: National Institute on Alcohol Abuse and Alcoholism.
Collections of the National Library of Medicine.

heroin's case, since, as Kaiko admitted, twice as much morphine had to be injected to get the equivalent results. As Cicely Saunders and Judith Quattlebaum had argued, addiction ought to be down-played as a consideration. It suggested that the WHO convention was a bankrupted approach – and the comfort level of the dying patient ought to be eased with fewer injections. Besides this, though, with heroin the physician would simply have "another arrow in the quiver" to be drawn upon when needed.[56]

Physicians, researchers, and pharmaceutical company representa-tives pressed the argument that heroin was less potent than Dilaudid, a synthetic opiate, and therefore an inferior option. Health and Human Services medical experts and their professional allies touted Dilaudid, manufactured by Knoll Pharmaceutical Company, as the safe, legal answer to the need for another high-potency narcotic for cancer pain. In 1982, Michael Grozier, MD, the vice-president of medical affairs at Knoll, contacted William F. Buckley to discuss his championing of Quattlebaum, CTIP, and the use of heroin for terminal cancer. According to Grozier, Buckley's assessment of the therapeutic use of heroin "misses the mark," had a "great many inconsistencies," and was off-base in its view of political sponsors.[57] The FDA seemed to agree and on 11 January 1984, it approved a high-potency for-mulation of hydromorphone named Dilaudid HP, stating at the time, "the drug will provide pain relief as great as can be obtained with any other narcotic including heroin, and can be delivered in a very small volume."[58] It was lauded as being more soluble and legal, but for pro-heroin supporters this pharmaceutical advancement was not "the ball game," so to speak.[59]

For others, though, the heated discussion over heroin in the mid-1980s masked questions about end-of-life care and served as a dis-traction. Dame Cicely Saunders, for example, who had founded the English hospice movement and popularized the use of heroin to help dying patients, felt that the American controversy was focusing atten-tion away from the larger issue, which was "the need to improve the general standard of care" in the United States. Similarly, Michael Levy, director of palliative care at the Fox Chase Cancer Center in Philadelphia, noted: "if the money and heat generated on the heroin bill were spent on developing new drugs and educating doctors on how to use the drugs we already have, patients would be a lot better off."[60] Dr Twycross chose not to engage in the American legislative process for the simple reason that the sanctioning of heroin in the

United States would not make a marked difference. Pain management and pain control in the US required an overhaul, so he chose to stay out of the fray.[61]

Apart from the argument over heroin's effectiveness, a fear also persisted that the drug would migrate from the hospital room to the streets. Representative Charlie Rangel (D-NY) established himself as a principal opponent of the legislation for precisely this reason. In a career that spanned over forty years (1971–present), Rangel, a charismatic and persuasive politician, spoke for the district of Harlem. The first black chairman of the House Ways and Means Committee, Rangel was also a founding member of the Congressional Black Caucus and during the 1980s served on the House Select Committee on Narcotics. He well understood that drugs themselves may embody racial and class-based meanings, as they become identified with specific segments of the population. This was certainly the case with opium and Asian Americans, marijuana and Hispanics, and crack cocaine and African Americans. Heroin, Rangel felt, was more likely to afflict his African-American constituents.

During his many years in office, he had taken strong stances on heroin and, more particularly, articulated the manifold dangers it held for his constituents, the majority of whom were African-American. In the early 1970s, many African-American political leaders and journalists, including Rangel, viewed the methadone maintenance program as an effort to "pacify, even stupefy, blacks."[62] According to Eric Schneider's *Smack*, it was widely believed amongst African Americans that methadone "took your manhood," "melted your bones," and was a "solution given to us by white, middle-class America." It was the "honky's way of keeping black men hooked."[63] In the words of one Black Panther leader, "We don't need the government making more *good* citizens. Methadone is just genocide, mostly against Black people." John Kaplan, writing in *The Hardest Drug*, described how methadone treatment was often called "drug enslavement."[64] For other commentators, "Addictive and deleterious substances have historically been used to further white interests."[65]

But in Rangel's view, the Compassionate Care Relief Act of 1984 was similar to methadone maintenance programs. Even though it called for a four-year window to study heroin for dying cancer patients, the bill represented a slippery slope towards heroin maintenance legislation – in short, the right of doctors to prescribe heroin to blacks in ghettos. Even worse, according to Arnold Trebach, Rangel interpreted the bill as an opening salvo for wholesale repeal of all the drug laws, the grand design of those who believed that enforcement had collapsed and was impossible to implement. This Rangel could not abide, for legalization would disproportionately affect the black population, especially those in his congressional district of Harlem.

> They're talking about my people. It's like saying "Let all those people who use heroin – it's a limited problem and only affects blacks, the minorities – let them have it. As long as they won't be bothering me ... Whether or not it destroys them, destroys their lives, that's not our problem."[66]

Rangel fought against the proposed law with great passion; he claimed that behind this bill were a lot of people who would soon openly advocate that "we just start legalizing the entire illicit drug manufacturing and transactions in the United States."[67] As a black Democrat with a sterling liberal record, Rangel's voice proved influential in the debate.

In an extraordinary twist of political circumstances of the kind that often accompanies complex policy matters, Rangel now found himself the subject of William F. Buckley's ire, a mandarin of the right-wing. In Buckley's view, Rangel was employing shoddy, sophomoric logic in addressing the legislation. "If heroin is bad, Rangel reasons, then why would Congress authorize its use. Well, Congress authorizes the use of napalm, and every day in every hospital, tools – and drugs – are used that, misused, would cause trouble, sometimes death."[68] In other words, Buckley was castigating Rangel for his conservative, unscientific, and race-based assessments of heroin for the dying. Moreover, other end-of-life drugs, including morphine and Dilaudid, were bought and sold on the streets and indeed preferred by many users. Medically pure Dilaudid, which went by the name "D," retailed at roughly $35 on various corners.[69] So how were they any safer?

Rangel's fears that heroin would leak out of hospitals and onto the streets of New York were shared by other lawmakers as well. Knowing this, supporters of the Compassionate Care Act devised clever sound-bites to manage this concern. For instance, during Arnold Trebach's testimony on 8 March 1984, he illustrated the amount of heroin needed for terminal patients, compared to the illegal quantities brought into the US annually:

I decided to place side by side, first, the highest amount of legal heroin that, I estimated, might be needed to treat all the cancer patients requiring it each year and, second, the lowest official estimate of the total amount of illicit heroin imported annually into this country. Those numbers were, first, 502 pounds of pure heroin and, second, 4.08 metric tons. Then I posited the worst-case scenario: assume all of the newly legal heroin were diverted and sold by criminals on the American black market. That diverted heroin would supply, at most, 5.6 percent of the illegal demand.[70]

In sum, the heroin that might slip out onto the streets of Harlem, as Rangel charged, was a relatively minor amount – not negligible, but small. Still, it took the Democratic representative from Michigan, John Dingell, to fully emphasize this point. During the floor debate, he underlined that four illegal tons of heroin are brought into this country each year," which was approximately "the weight of two elephants." Medical use for dying cancer patients, said Dingell sharply, would be "a pimple on the posterior of one of those elephants."[71] According to Henry Waxman, who adopted more grandiose language, the Compassionate Pain Relief Act might act as a starting point for "a compassionate, balanced, and hopeful drug policy for this nation."[72]

To counter this point, opponents employed language that conflated the scientific assessments and medical applications of heroin with fears of drug abuse and addiction. In particular, the susceptibility of young people to heroin was underscored. The response from the National Federation of Parents for Drug Free Youth, for example, outlined that the Compassionate Pain Relief Act would validate heroin, and "to falsely legitimize heroin sends the wrong message about this devastating and illegal drug to our youth."[73] Even more boldly, Hamilton Fish Jr (R-NY), Charles Rangel's colleague from New York, proclaimed: "This bill will send a signal to the youth of this nation that 'heroin is ok.'" It was an argument that harkened back to nearly fifteen years earlier, when *Time* magazine had as its cover story "Kids and Heroin: The Adolescent Epidemic."[74]

As the presidential and congressional elections approached in 1984, the argument against heroin proved persuasive. On 18 September 1984, the Act was decisively defeated in the House of Representatives, 355 to 55. Afterward, Henry Waxman recounted how many of his colleagues did not doubt the medical value of heroin, nor did they worry about the minuscule amount that could be diverted to the streets. Instead, Waxman's colleagues noted that a vote in favour of the bill enabled their opponents in the forthcoming election to label them as "heroin pushers."[75]

THE END OF THE 1980S

Quattlebaum finally ceased operations at the National Committee for the Treatment of Intractable Pain in 1989, fifteen years after co-founding the organization. During that time, she clearly helped advance the dialogue about palliative care treatment in American society, as well as the proper approach to drug policy. Against the backdrop of a War on Drugs, she failed on several occasions to legislate the controlled use of heroin in hospices and beyond; the bill was revived again in 1987–88, only to stall out once more; still, according to William F. Buckley Jr, it was a "very long fight, and Judith Quattlebaum of Washington has led it unflaggingly."[76] She successfully collaborated with the scientific community, with cancer advocates, and with politicians, and influenced the legislative process.

In 1988, Quattlebaum articulated concerns about the failure of her mission as co-founder of CTIP and what that suggested in the years ahead. She criticized the medical community for its failure "to rethink its myths and prejudices" about suffering terminal cancer patients, which, in turn, "has helped maintain myths among the public." In her view, heroin was not a panacea at all; rather, the effort to make heroin available was a "limited goal and a partial solution," and she did not claim it would solve all the problems associated with terminal cancer pain. She believed, moreover, that the debate about heroin's use in a controlled setting exposed crucial "processes" which had led to the hospice movement in the first place and ultimately hindered other solutions in end-of-life care. On the one hand, she insisted that there was widespread denial that pain existed and still a strong reluctance to position the patient's pain at the centre of care. On the other hand, she underlined how an unjustified panic about narcotics for those same patients was accompanied by narrow-mindedness in the American medical establishment, as well as in the Department of Health and Human Services, the Drug Enforcement Administration, and the American Medical Association.[77]

While Reagan administration officials, along with the American Medical Association and anti-drug groups, resisted the use of heroin as a therapy for cancer patients, the policy nevertheless received sympathetic consideration from many conservatives and liberals, Republicans and Democrats. The argument, overall, was one in which moral considerations and ethical formulations bled into the calculations involved in crime prevention, consumer protection, and evidence-based policy-making. More than that, heroin therapy prompted questions about the proper treatment of pain and the rights of dying patients in palliative care, not just in hospices but in hospitals and individual homes as well. By the mid-1980s, the hospice movement had logged victories, grown, and charted a new course in the treatment of dying Americans. In the ensuing drama over heroin treatment, the benevolent values of this movement clashed with proponents of anti-drug agendas.

These were all elements of the contemporaneous Canadian discussion, of course. Quattlebaum and Dr Gifford-Jones produced very similar arguments. Since the 1960s, palliative care had developed and spread in both Canada and the United States. Law enforcement officials in both countries resisted heroin's legalization, in any form. Yet, several issues generated different outcomes. The first was that the Canadian Medical Association eventually demonstrated limited support of heroin, while a second crucial difference was the lack of any meaningful racial element in the Canadian legislative calculations. There was no equivalent of Charlie Rangel in Canada, nor was there an explicit War on Drugs launched by the Liberals or Conservatives. Concerns about crime were present in each debate, although Conservatives opted to reject the previous government's heroin plan *and* the link between heroin and dangers to the public good. Finally, the influence of the British medical system on Canada was certainly influential.

In the US, health activists who touted the patient's right to select his or her type of pain medication met resistance from the Reagan administration, which was prosecuting its War on Drugs and promoting regulatory reform for the pharmaceutical industry. Future scholars will need to explore the role of market calculations and the role of drug-makers in impacting the American policy. New studies of Purdue Pharma and articles in the *New England Journal of Medicine* help us understand the current opioid crisis, and it would be valuable to explore heroin in palliative care too. If there was an emerging junk equation at the end of the 1980s, the fluctuating scientific, political, and moral variables made it – as Judith Quattlebaum could surely attest – incredibly difficult to solve.

LAETRILE'S LIFE CYCLE AFTER
THE DEATH OF STEVE MCQUEEN

In the 2013 movie *Dallas Buyers Club*, we are exposed to valiant patient activism during the 1980s AIDS crisis in the United States. Based on the true story of Ron Woodroof, a hard-partying and homophobic Texas tradesman, the film shows a remarkably thin Matthew McConaughey battle his sickness and inner demons, as well as the drug industry and government. Woodroof, who's unhappy with his illegally purchased zidovudine, known as AZT, and on the edge of death, seeks out alternative and experimental drugs from a doctor in Mexico. Being the savvy entrepreneur and hustler that he is, Woodroof quickly establishes a club (charging a $400 membership fee) to sell his smuggled wares, including vitamins, DDC, and Peptide T. In doing so, he runs afoul of the Food and Drug Administration and the Drug Enforcement Administration and is essentially forced to confront the existing power structure of drug regulation.

At one point in the film, Woodroof storms a town hall meeting of citizens, drug company leaders, and FDA regulators and, while still attached to his IV bag, starts finger-pointing. "People are dying. And y'all up there are afraid that we're gonna find an alternative without you." Inevitably, bums shift in chairs. Chests are puffed up. And murmurs echo in the room. "You see," Ron continues, "the pharma companies pay the FDA to push their product. They don't want to see my research. I don't have enough cash in my pocket to make it worth their while." The message is not difficult to discern. Overly cautious and slow, as well as a pawn of the pharmaceutical industry, the FDA is portrayed as the black hat to Woodroof's rugged anti-hero. The FDA is characterized as brutally uncaring and, for some conservative commentators, this helps expose the agency for what it is – a sclerotic, centralized bureaucracy unable to respond to the AIDS crisis.

The film revealed a lot about drug regulation in the late 1970s and 1980s. It was a time when the regulation of Big Pharma got twisted, turned, and pulled upside down by politicians, consumer groups, and drug industry leaders. Of course, at the centre of the tug-of-war was the FDA, an independent government agency under constant pressure. The AIDS crisis raised the stakes even higher: for people such as Ron Woodroof who needed special, experimental HIV/AIDS drugs, and for regulators, who sought to carry out their duties in a professional manner. Tough decisions about access to drugs were necessary. Was the FDA perfect? Certainly not. But was the FDA a cardboard villain, as the movie suggests? No.[1]

Much of the film depicts AZT as dangerously toxic and perhaps worse than the sickness it was meant to cure. Woodroof takes the drug at the beginning of the film, reacts poorly, and thereafter tells his club members to dump their supply. Ron Woodroof even physically assaults a doctor at Texas Mercy Hospital for administering AZT to his friend Rayon (played by Jared Leto), who dies shortly thereafter. "Murderer," shouts Ron, "murderer." The problem with this depiction, of course, is that AZT was actually a rather effective therapy for HIV/AIDS, although the dosages were far too high during the initial trials. The reason behind this was simple: physicians were concerned a lower dose wouldn't be enough to slow the virus. They wanted to hit it hard. Knock it out. Still, the dosage issue wasn't properly addressed in the film and was only given a brief moment, when Dr Eve Saks (played by Jennifer Garner) quietly orders that her patients receive a smaller dosage. Just as important, AZT was used not in combination therapy but instead on its own. It wasn't until the mid-1990s that researchers and physicians started using a cocktail of antivirals. This became known as highly active antiretroviral therapy (HAART), which helped transform HIV from a full-on death sentence into a chronic and manageable disease.[2]

Woodroof, of course, didn't have all the answers. Many of the drugs that his club imported from Mexico and provided to its members were useless. For instance, Peptide T: Woodroof used it regularly and was a massive advocate, despite the fact that the research community found it to be ineffective (although not harmful) and it was never approved. Another example was Compound Q, a drug linked to a number of deaths during clinical trials. This prompted the FDA to crack down on the drug, and, indeed, most buyers' clubs across the country pulled it, except for Woodroof's. While he was on the cutting edge of research and willing to challenge conventional wisdom, he was still fallible.[3]

The FDA was also misrepresented, considering it didn't fight tooth-and-nail with AIDS groups and buyers' clubs. Near the end of the movie, a judge in California criticizes the FDA and its unwillingness to allow HIV/AIDS patients to have access to Peptide T. According to the judge, "the FDA was formed to protect people, not prevent them from getting help." One could be forgiven for thinking that the agency was obstructing sick Americans on a regular basis. Yet, the agency was anything but viciously cold-hearted or adversarial toward HIV/AIDS patients. With minimal direction from the slow-moving Reagan administration, the FDA cooperated with underground AIDS drug trials, included AIDS movement leaders in policy discussions, and was generally tolerant of buyers' clubs. Numerous scholars, including myself, have contended that AIDS activists proved very successful at bending the FDA to their will, a fact noticeably absent in *Dallas Buyers Club*. Tough choices still had to be made, of course, but the FDA was far from immovable. The same judge who criticized the FDA also opined, "The law doesn't seem to make common sense sometimes. If a person is found to be terminally ill, well they ought to be able to take just about anything they feel will help … but that's not the law."[4]

This debate was not altogether new. The story of Laetrile, much like *Dallas Buyers Club*, highlights the tricky line that separates consumer protection and product innovation, the right to choose one's medicine, and the state's obligation to protect citizens from specious drugs. Caught in a middle ground between opposing factions and heterogeneous stakeholders was the FDA, as I argued in my first book. Historical actors and groups on both the left and right of the socio-political spectrum – consumer advocates, regulatory reformers, academicians, industry representatives, and administration officials – sought to spread the idea that regulations governing the nation's drug supply were insufficient. Numerous groups regarded the agency as an inefficient entity, whereas others viewed the agency as an extension of Big Pharma. The FDA, a prisoner of disenchantment with government and American institutions, was compelled to negotiate these contrary pressures, even as the number of congressional hearings increased. For some American critics on the right, it was intolerable that an Eastern Bloc autocrat such as

Marshal Tito in the former Yugoslavia should have access to new drugs before American consumers. Libertarians declared that individuals in a genuinely free society must be permitted – allowed – to take any medicine they wished. According to this logic, government had zero responsibility for regulating drugs in the first place.[5]

Regulatory reformers in the 1970s impugned government. They saw the FDA as a "hidebound, bureaucratic morass."[6] Dr Louis Lasagna, of Rochester University's Medical School and an expert on the drug approval process who tilted toward less regulation, told Congress in 1978: "I have been increasingly alarmed over the past several years at the disastrous effects FDA regulations and their administration have had on drug research and development in this country."[7] Another regulatory reformer, Congressman James Scheuer (D-NY), chairman of the Oversight Committee of the Committee on Science and Technology, held that consumer activism stifled industry. "How far behind we were in the sophisticated expeditious approval of a new drug," he contended, was a serious problem that needed immediate investigation.[8] Dr William Wardell, a conspicuous critic of the FDA who actually invented the "drug lag" phrase, sought a drug approval process that was devoid of red tape.[9]

In reply to such analyses, FDA chief Dr Donald Kennedy shot back. He declared that the "drug lag" term was useless in resolving the agency's perceived drug approval problem. All of the derisive talk amounted to *brutum fulmen*, or senseless thunderbolts. The big picture mattered more. To this end, in July 1979, Kennedy outlined a number of problems that contributed to the length of time to approve a drug, which included the public's role in the process, the stringent requirements for human subjects, and several others. He also offered some solutions. Kennedy emphasized that it was important to think about "whether we in the United States have been approving drugs as rapidly as we can, given the system of regulation established by law." The commissioner later admitted, "the answer to that question, is that we are now approaching the maximum rate possible commensurate with the design of the system itself."[10] This was something of an admission, to be fair.

Laetrile, which was promoted as a cancer treatment in the 1970s and proved one of the most popular alternative medicines in decades, crystallized debates about consumer choice, government intrusion, and the availability of drugs. It took a strange trip. Laetrile embodied the growing influence of such interest groups as the Center for

Science in the Public Interest and Public Citizen, who competed fiercely with such organizations as the Pharmaceutical Research and Manufacturers Association (phRMA), the Heritage Foundation, and the American Enterprise Institute. The drug represented how, at different times, the FDA has rebranded itself as a "regulatory agency," a "law enforcement agency," or a "science agency," depending on the political party in power and the philosophy of its commissioner.[11]

For Gerald E. Markle and James C. Peterson, "[a]t the core of the Laetrile movement" were "a few small organizations devoted" to its promotion. These organizations used tenets of the natural and alternative health movements of the 1960s, as well as playing up the failings of government and long-standing medical institutions.[12] *Science* was less forgiving, suggesting that Laetrile was bound up in the quest for "nonrational and simplistic remedies for ailments both physical and spiritual, as manifested through interest in the occult, faith healing, astrology, UFO's, and so forth."[13] According to *Time* magazine, by 1976 Laetrile had attracted "an avid, almost evangelical band of followers," a group that included members of the "right-wing John Birch society," an ultraconservative group that pushed back against Communist infiltration and expanding government. These supporters viewed the FDA's ban on Laetrile as "a restraint on individual freedom."[14]

"THE FLAG OF MEDICAL FREEDOM"

As we saw in previous chapters, the dispute over cancer, heroin, and end-of-life care roused such passion because it linked cancer, the most dreaded disease of the 1970s and early 1980s, with heroin, the most feared drug of the era.[15] According to James Patterson, "The history of cancer in America is also a history of social and cultural tensions. Set against the optimistic anticancer alliance were a variety of people, many of them relatively poor and ill-educated." These Americans, he argued, together constituted "what I call a cancer counterculture, skeptical about orthodox medical notions of disease and about the claims to expert knowledge by what they came to call the Cancer Establishment." Some of these cynics relied on home remedies, others on quackery or traditional and folk wisdom, while others used religious faith. "The counterculture," Patterson wrote, "clashed often with the confident, optimistic allies against cancer. Indeed, the tension between the two groups illustrates durable social and cultural divisions in modern America."[16]

Laetrile – basically an extraction of a chemical called amygdalin – was the embodiment of that tension. It was a means to address cancer in the mid-1970s and 1980s. The scientific guru behind Laetrile was Ernst T. Krebs Jr, a biochemist whose father, a doctor, first propounded the idea that apricot pits had anticancer properties. The junior Krebs (who later became the scientific director of the Committee for Freedom of Choice in Medicine) refined the "formula" in the late 1940s and gave it the name Laetrile. Krebs's theory was that cancer cells had large quantities of an enzyme called beta-glycosidase, which released the hydrogen cyanide in the amygdalin to kill the cells. He hypothesized that normal cells were not affected because they possessed another enzyme, rhodenase, which detoxified the cyanide. Laetrile can be found all over the globe, in such foods as chickpeas, lentils, lima beans, cashews, barley, brown rice, and apricot pits. (For commercial purposes, Laetrile was often extracted from apricot and peach pits.) During the 1950s and 1960s, physicians employed Laetrile in combination therapies for cancer, even as it faced resistance from the mainstream medical establishment and struggled with "an aura of illegality."[17] This was the case because, quite simply, as agreeable as Krebs's ideas were, and as much as cancer patients craved an alternative, "natural" medicine, Laetrile's effectiveness was not confirmed by any scientific research.

The safety and efficacy of Laetrile grew into a larger point of contestation among members of Congress, the FDA, physician organizations, medical institutes, and patient-consumer groups. In many ways, the debate over this treatment embodied questions of scientific and medical authority that had troubled the FDA since its inception, although it was also a reflection of Laetrile's unusually powerful combination of followers and advocates. The dispute began as early as the early 1960s, when such individuals as Krebs and McNaughton administered the chemical to patients outside the law. Andrew R.L. McNaughton, an English-born Canadian "adventurer" and Laetrile researcher/entrepreneur, was especially influential. He would have protracted legal battles in California, with the FDA, and in 1963–64 the Canadian Food and Drug Directorate barred any further distribution of Laetrile on the basis that its safety and efficacy had not been established.

Ever resourceful, McNaughton continued to successfully manoeuvre within a climate of illegality, convince others about his cause, and create a foundation of legitimacy. On the one hand, he recruited former National Cancer Institute scientist Dean Burk, who provided a "recognizable voice with credentials from government service and in professional medicine," and offered lamentations about the FDA's approach to cancer and clinical experiment.[18] Having worked with Laetrile at the NCI, Burk was mostly sensible in his public statements, which included references to the use of Laetrile in other jurisdictions, as well as its therapeutic potential. On the other hand, McNaughton, among others, fostered a network of interest groups, such as the International Association of Cancer Victims and Friends and Cancer Control Society – both of which espoused naturopathic, homeopathic language and critiqued "out-of-date, out-moded, so-called 'orthodox' treatment."[19] Unlike Burk, members of these groups often possessed conspiratorial views, identified with neo-conservative beliefs, and castigated the FDA for its unwillingness to allow further research into Laetrile.

In 1970, McNaughton moved from Montreal to California and created a non-profit scientific research organization called the McNaughton Foundation. He soon submitted to the FDA an Investigational New Drug (IND) application to study Laetrile. His application was ultimately rejected, since it was determined by the FDA that the preclinical evidence failed to demonstrate Laetrile might be effective as an anti-cancer agent – in other words, there was a lack of evidence in support of the study. This did not stop him, though. He was instrumental in having G.D. Kittler's pro-Laetrile articles published in the US and then relocated to Tijuana, Mexico, where he established manufacturing and treatment facilities. According to historian James Harvey Young, this new base just across the border acted as a transshipment point for Laetrile and also a flagship treatment centre. "The first patient treated in Tijuana created the International Association of Cancer Victims and Friends, which publicized Laetrile, helped cancer patients visit Mexico, and fly the flag of medical freedom."[20] Supporters of Laetrile also established the Cancer Control Society, which proved surprisingly successful in getting the message out to the middle class.

Their message aligned well with conservative views about infringements on American freedom, as well as anti-government sentiments, growing patient-consumer activism, and therapeutic individualism.[21] According to a review by the National Cancer Institute (NCI), McNaughton and his devotees viewed the FDA's early rejection as an attempt by the US government to block access to new,

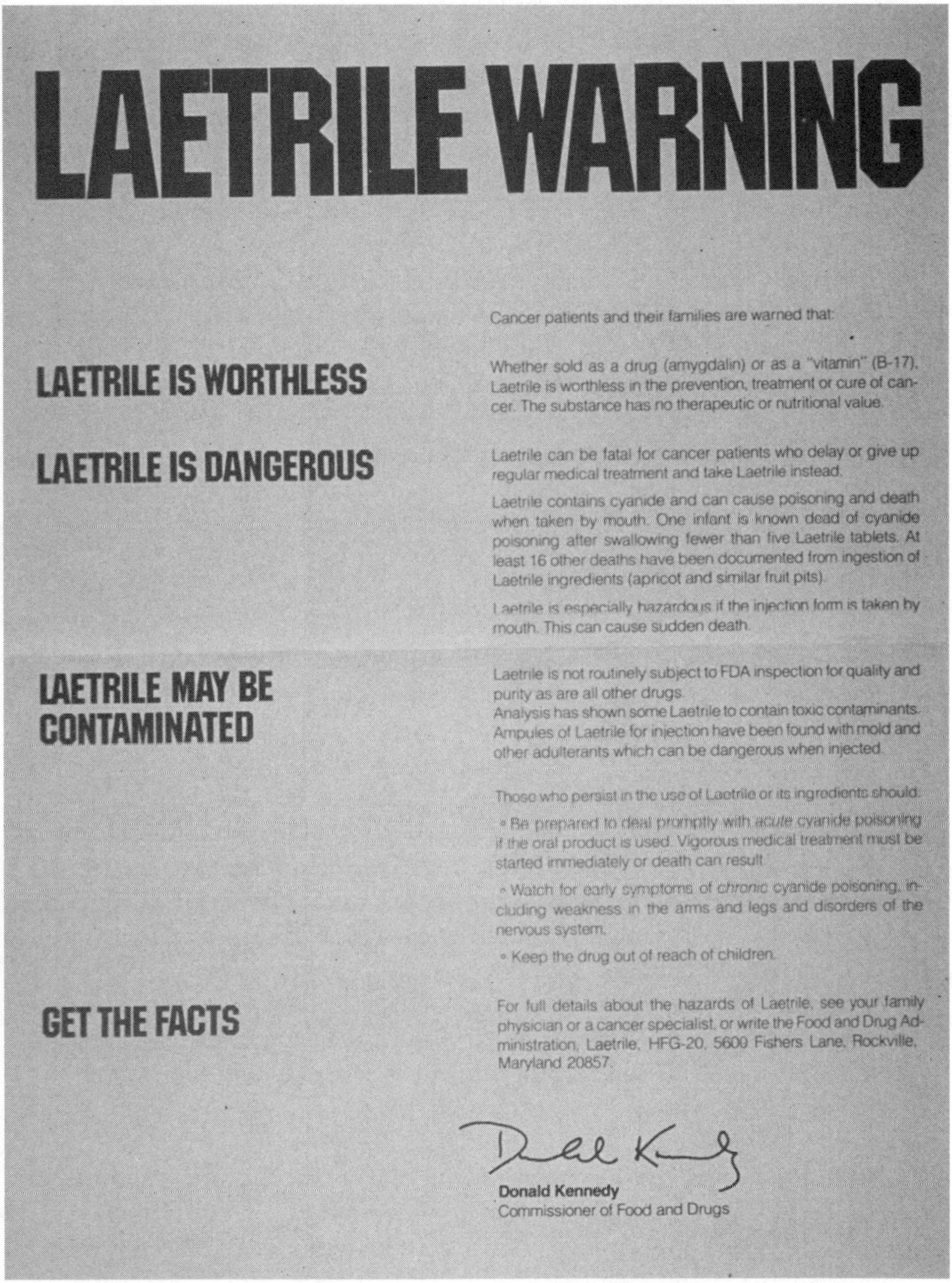

LAETRILE WARNING

Cancer patients and their families are warned that:

LAETRILE IS WORTHLESS

Whether sold as a drug (amygdalin) or as a "vitamin" (B-17), Laetrile is worthless in the prevention, treatment or cure of cancer. The substance has no therapeutic or nutritional value.

LAETRILE IS DANGEROUS

Laetrile can be fatal for cancer patients who delay or give up regular medical treatment and take Laetrile instead.

Laetrile contains cyanide and can cause poisoning and death when taken by mouth. One infant is known dead of cyanide poisoning after swallowing fewer than five Laetrile tablets. At least 16 other deaths have been documented from ingestion of Laetrile ingredients (apricot and similar fruit pits).

Laetrile is especially hazardous if the injection form is taken by mouth. This can cause sudden death.

LAETRILE MAY BE CONTAMINATED

Laetrile is not routinely subject to FDA inspection for quality and purity as are all other drugs.
Analysis has shown some Laetrile to contain toxic contaminants. Ampules of Laetrile for injection have been found with mold and other adulterants which can be dangerous when injected.

Those who persist in the use of Laetrile or its ingredients should:

- Be prepared to deal promptly with *acute* cyanide poisoning if the oral product is used. Vigorous medical treatment must be started immediately or death can result.
- Watch for early symptoms of *chronic* cyanide poisoning, including weakness in the arms and legs and disorders of the nervous system.
- Keep the drug out of reach of children.

GET THE FACTS

For full details about the hazards of Laetrile, see your family physician or a cancer specialist, or write the Food and Drug Administration, Laetrile, HFG-20, 5600 Fishers Lane, Rockville, Maryland 20857.

Donald Kennedy
Commissioner of Food and Drugs

FIGURE 3.1 "Laetrile Warning." The poster was circulated across the United States. Rockville, MD: Food and Drug Administration, 1977. Collections of the National Library of Medicine.

promising cancer therapies, and pressure mounted to make Laetrile available to the public. In California, physician John A. Richardson, who was also a member of the ultraconservative John Birch Society, was arrested and prosecuted for prescribing Laetrile under the state's anti-quackery laws; unfortunately, two trials ended with hung juries before California's Board of Medical Quality Assurance intervened and revoked Richardson's licence. Similar to Ron Woodroof in Texas, Richardson was politically conservative and, along with his supporters, adopted a libertarian position regarding freedom of choice in health care, and in the medical marketplace more specifically.[22]

It was positioned in a longer historical framework as well, with Laetrile leaders cleverly using the Founding Fathers of the United States to underscore concepts of therapeutic autonomy. At the outset of a retrospective 1980 paper, "The Laetrile Phenomenon," Robert W. Bradford and Michael Culbert used Dr Benjamin Rush, who served as the first US Surgeon General and signed the Declaration of Independence, to emphasize their point that Laetrile's unavailability pointed to broader systemic problems in health care and the country more broadly. "The Constitution of this republic," wrote Rush in 1776, "should make special provisions for medical freedom as well as religious freedom." "To restrict the art of healing to one class of men and deny equal privilege to another," he argued, was "un-American and despotic." That this use of Rush was devoid of both nuance and context seemed lost on Bradford and Culbert. It was shoddy, and certainly *ipse dixit*, meaning that the assertion rested on the authority of Rush and not the evidence. But it bolstered the notion that Laetrile represented a "new idea," confronted the "medical status quo," and served as a "harbinger of [a] fullscale revolution in medicine."[23]

One of the key figures supporting Laetrile and the movement buttressing the therapy was journalist Michael Culbert. Naturally personable, easy to laugh, and quick to banter, the Kansas-born Culbert developed a reputation for not only a razor-sharp mind but also an ability to make others feel comfortable. In the 1970s as a reporter for the *Berkeley Daily Gazette*, he covered the trial of Dr John Richardson, who was being prosecuted for treating cancer patients with Laetrile. Culbert was seemingly convinced by Richardson's position, and he later described how strange political bedfellows were created in this atmosphere of alternative therapy. For instance, Culbert recalled how "I would go to the Berkeley municipal court ... and there were McGovern-for-president left-wing hippies in the audience who were in favour of this John Birch doctor."[24] Laetrile was an "issue that was far beyond left and right ... The freedom-of-choice movement was a populist revolution." As an organizer and propagandist, he founded the Committee for Freedom of Choice in Cancer Therapy, Inc., and later the Committee for Freedom of Choice in Medicine, as well as the International Council for Health Freedom. According to Ralph Moss, another stalwart in the alternative medicine movement and author of a pro-Laetrile book, Culbert "had an enormous influence on the course of cancer treatment, although that influence will never be acknowledged in the standard sources."[25]

By 1976, Culbert's medical and business interests had grown tremendously, consisting of roughly 450 chapters around the country and a membership of 23,000, which included 800 doctors and Representative Larry P. MacDonald (D-GA), a urologist who had treated many patients with Laetrile. That year, the committee held several symposia where its chairman, Robert William Bradford (who had been indicted for Laetrile smuggling), provided courses on the role of diet and nutrition in the treatment of degenerative diseases. The committee also conducted open meetings for the general public around the country which, according to Culbert, attracted anywhere from a couple of dozen to over a thousand people.[26] It helped, too, that everyone involved was writing a book to communicate the pro-Laetrile agenda. Richardson produced *Laetrile Case Histories*, Kittler published *Laetrile: Control for Cancer*, and Culbert wrote *Freedom from Cancer* and *Vitamin B 17: Forbidden Weapon of Cancer*. Laetrile became big business. Investigations by Californian authorities, for example, exposed the huge sums of money that Laetrile leaders were squirrelling away in the bank, estimated in the millions.

Yet, none of this would have been possible without the "rights revolution" of the 1970s and the changing information environment, which ran parallel to and reinforced the alternative health care movement. By the late 1960s and early 1970s, widespread political activist movements focused on the Vietnam War, civil rights for African Americans, Native American Indians, and Latin Americans, and the elevation of second-wave feminism. "Patients' rights" also emerged in this milieu, and the genesis point often referred to was the drafting in 1970 of twenty-six such rights by the National Welfare Rights Organization, which later led to the American Hospital Association's "Patient's Bill of Rights" in 1973. These were momentous in that they declared, unequivocally, that a patient has the right to refuse treatment, but also to "obtain from his physician complete current information concerning his diagnosis, treatment, and prognosis, in terms the patient can be reasonably expected to understand."[27] Even as "patients' rights" grew in strength, the 1970s heralded a change in the amount of medical information available to citizens in the medical marketplace, information from sources such as the pro-Laetrile books *Freedom from Cancer* and *Laetrile: Control for Cancer*. For much of the history of what we would now call patient safety and "patients' rights," advocacy by patients was set in the context of the consumer movement, and focused primarily on public perceptions of unsafe medical practices, insufficient accountability, and lack of openness. Events such as the 1975 Congressional hearings on unnecessary surgery and ABC's 1982 "The Deep Sleep" special on anesthesia mortality, for instance, fashioned the backdrop for activist groups such as Charles Inlander's People's Medical Society, the Center for Medical Consumers, and the Public Citizen's Health Research Group, all of which tried to impact regulation and provide medical information to the public.

Today, the vaccine skeptic Jenny McCarthy best embodies the patient-consumer who challenges the medical establishment, defies conventional wisdom, and champions alternative approaches to treatment. In her well-publicized exploits, McCarthy has promoted the idea that vaccines cause autism and that chelation therapy helped cure her son of autism. Both claims are unsupported by medical consensus, yet the fact that she empowered herself by going onto the internet, discovering new treatments, and essentially standing athwart orthodox medical practices ingratiated her to many people. "Fighting Autism with My Son" and "How I Saved My Son" are eye-catching banners, although Paul Offit has explained in *Autism's False Prophets* that high drama, heroic headlines, charismatic personalities, conspiracy theories, and accusations – bolstered by freely available medical information – undermine public health.[28]

With the Laetrile movement, as in the case of the anti-vaccine movement, much of the underlying ethos had to do with disenchantment with the relative failures of conventional therapy and a perception that not enough was being done. In *World without Cancer: The Story of Vitamin B-17*, for example, G. Edward Griffin argued that standard cancer therapy – radiation, surgery, and chemotherapy – was a shambles. It not only failed to achieve notable remission rates but resulted in a significant reduction in quality of life. More than that, the book argued that policy-makers in the medical, pharmaceutical, research, and fund-raising organizations deliberately or unconsciously strove not to "prevent and cure cancer in order to perpetuate their functions."[29] This type of anti-establishment, "us vs. them" reasoning was prevalent in many pro-Laetrile groups, just as it was epitomized in Ron Woodroof's *Dallas Buyers Club* or in Jenny McCarthy's vaccine hesitancy. It certainly didn't help that some physicians pushed back hard – and rather patronizingly, too – against patient-consumer agency and choice in the medical sphere. While debating Laetrile, Dr Crippen suggested in the pages of the *Hastings Center Report* that "[i]t is unfortunate but true that the lay public are not intelligent, informed consumers when it comes to health care. They do not have the expertise to evaluate critically drugs or methods of care. Like it or not, they are at our mercy."[30]

A FOOTBALL

The *New England Journal of Medicine* called the discussion "Laetrilomania" and the compound quickly became a political football. Public opinion was divided and lawmakers, much like in the case of medical heroin, were bombarded with letters supporting Laetrile.[31] Of course, advocates for Laetrile claimed variously that the substance was effective in the cure or mitigation of cancer, prevented cancer, promoted the action of other cancer therapies, was an analgesic, and had value in the treatment of sickle cell anemia, parasitic disease, and hypertension. Unfortunately, none of these properties of Laetrile was ever demonstrated in a controlled investigation, and experts from the American Cancer Society, the American Medical Association, and the Committee on Neoplastic Diseases of the American Academy of Pediatrics largely did not acknowledge it as effective. In the November-December 1977 issue of the agency's *Drug Bulletin*, distributed to over a million health care workers in the United States, the outright rejection of Laetrile was unmistakable. It had the potential to "cause poisoning and death when taken by mouth," the article read, and was not subject to FDA inspections.[32] Moreover, in a relatively unusual move, the agency sent 10,000 posters across the US to spread awareness about Laetrile's toxicity and unregulated nature. From the FDA's perspective, scant anecdotal evidence supported the use of Laetrile, and after an extensive five-month review the agency deemed there was insufficient scientific proof to justify its use at all. The agency called it "worthless and illegal as a cancer remedy."[33]

Still, multiple court cases across the United States challenged the government's authority in determining which drugs should be available to cancer patient-consumers, and the result was that Laetrile was legalized in twenty-four states by October 1982, although the majority passed legislation between 1977 and 1979. The provisions of these state bills were incredibly diverse, as some protected physicians and pharmacists, while others did not. Some specified that written records were to be filed and reviewed, and some of the laws required a prescription, whereas others did not. In short, the Laetrile laws – passed in places such as Alaska and Arizona, Oklahoma and Oregon – were wildly variable. Similarly, customs officials in San Diego were seizing 40,000 three-gram vials of Laetrile every month, roughly fifteen thousand Americans were seeking Laetrile treatments in Mexico, and an estimated 70,000 Americans had already used Laetrile.[34]

Meanwhile, US Representative Steven D. Symms (R-ID) sought to legalize Laetrile nationally and curtail the authority of the FDA. A long-time critic of the FDA, Symms propounded a growing view that bureaucrats in the agency lacked compassion for patients – essentially that there was too much emotional distance between FDA officers and patient-consumers.[35] First elected in 1972, Symms was both "upbeat and friendly," as well as a showman with a talent for grabbing headlines. (Besides his criticisms of drug regulation, for example, he once turned up at an anti–gun control news conference packing two revolvers.) In 1977, Symms responded to "grass roots support" and "outrage over the Laetrile situation," as he put it, when he sponsored federal legislation called the "Medical Freedom of Choice Bill."[36] The issue, as in the case of gun control, was freedom. "The American people should be allowed to make their own decisions. They shouldn't have the bureaucrats in Washington, D.C. trying to decide for them."[37]

As Symms put it, the bill expedited new pharmaceutical drugs to market, including Laetrile. Not proven inherently harmful, yet unavailable for doctors and patients either. "My bill would make Laetrile available to physicians who want to use it ... and if there is nothing to it, we'll find out in a hurry."[38] Interestingly, one of the unintended consequences of the bill was its influence on discussions of marijuana. Under Symms's legislation, the FDA had the authority to make marijuana available in drugstores if it determined its controlled use was not dangerous. Symms, being opposed to cannabis, was forced to address this issue and asserted that the FDA would not likely certify marijuana safe – because of both scientific and political uncertainties. "It would have to be an awful wild fluke," he told reporters. In Ronald Reagan, Symms found a vocal supporter. During a radio address, Reagan described the law as a "pro-consumer, anti-monopoly" measure, and one that returned decision-making authority to physicians. "Doctors have displayed, over the years, a great ability to sort out medicines which aren't very effective," noted Reagan, and Symms's efforts would amend the "hasty, panic-inspired" laws of the 1962 thalidomide tragedy, which "hardly benefited the American people."[39] And while Symms was able to attract 110 cosponsors, and though half the states passed legalization statutes, his "Medical Freedom of Choice Bill" died by the early 1980s.[40]

Meanwhile, at the state level, in 1977 various efforts were taken to bypass federal regulations that prohibited the sale of drugs with unproved medicinal values, including Laetrile. In such places as Indiana and Oregon, lawmakers and health officials challenged the FDA and federal health regulations. In Indiana, saccharin was legalized, whereas in Oregon DMSO (dimethyl sulfoxide) was legalized. Authorities in Nevada approved the manufacture and sale of the anti-aging Gerovital, even though many in the scientific community and at the FDA disagreed. Running parallel with Symm's championing of Laetrile, these moves suggested more than long-standing states' rights considerations. These laws marked a growing trend against consumer protection and excessive governmental regulation, as well as therapeutic freedom of choice in the medical marketplace. Efforts appeared more personal for others. In voting in favour of a Laetrile bill, Arizona Representative Sam McConnell was pleased to "tell the FDA to go fly a kite."[41]

In pushing back against the state laws and the freedom argument made by Symms, Culbert, and their associates, the physician David Crippen adopted a big-picture approach:

In our society, we have defined limits over which the freedoms of the individual may not extend. The freedoms of the individual are subservient to the rights and ultimate well-being of the group. Thus, I may not yell "fire" in a crowded theater and call it freedom of speech. If we, as responsible physicians, allow demonstratably ineffective drugs on the market without a fight, a great number of people who simply don't know any better will get worthless, expensive hoaxes instead of effective treatment.[42]

Legal wrangling, consumer activism, and the lack of scientific data and consensus prolonged the debate over Laetrile. In 1977, for instance, a federal district judge in Oklahoma named Luther Bohanon ruled that terminally ill cancer patients could obtain a personal supply of Laetrile as long they signed an affidavit.[43] Senator Edward Kennedy (D-MA) held hearings in 1977 in which Laetrile promoters declared that a collection of organizations, including the FDA, AMA, NCI, and American Cancer Society (as well as the Rockefeller family), conspired against Laetrile. Kennedy, who said he would champion Laetrile in the Senate if a positive and reproducible clinical trial was concluded, nevertheless regarded the Laetrile advocates "with a blend of amusement and contempt." He also worried they offered cancer patients "a false sense of hope."[44] By 1978, it was estimated that between 50,000 and 100,000 were taking over 1 million milligrams a month.[45] In 1979, the FDA's resistance to the drug was vindicated when the Supreme Court rejected the arguments made by the proponents of Laetrile and upheld existing food and drug statutes, including the 1962 law. The unanimous decision stated:

> Since the turn of the century, resourceful entrepreneurs have advertised a wide variety of purportedly simple and painless cures for cancer, including lineaments of turpentine, mustard, oil, eggs, and ammonia; peat moss; arrangements of colored floodlights; pastes made from glycerin and limburger cheese; mineral tablets; and "Fountain of Youth" mixtures of spices, oil and suet … Congress could reasonably have determined to protect the terminally ill, no less than other patients, from the vast range of self-styled panaceas that inventive minds can devise.[46]

Even with this decision, researchers and medical doctors operated in an environment in which definitive studies and answers about Laetrile were largely absent. Put simply, doubts remained. To rectify this, the National Cancer Institute grew more involved. The director of the NCI, Frank Rauscher, had stated rather definitively in 1976, "I wish it worked, but … it simply is not active against cancer."[47] In 1978, though, the NCI initiated a retrospective case review (a study of past cases) and sent over 400,000 letters to doctors and other practitioners, asking them to submit positive results from cases involving Laetrile. In response, the NCI received only 93 "positive" evaluations – and only 6 of those had evidence of significant tumour shrinkage.[48]

Thereafter, the NCI, given the widespread interest and the long, bitter dispute within the scientific community and activist community, further tested Laetrile in 1980. The tests, which included 178 patients with advanced cancer, were conducted in four major medical centres (the Mayo Clinic, University of California Los Angeles, University of Arizona Health Sciences Center, and Memorial Sloan-Kettering) and the unfavourable results were presented in April 1981. At that year's annual meeting of the American Society for Clinical Oncology, the director of the NCI, Dr Vincent DeVita Jr, pronounced, "The findings present public evidence of Laetrile's failure as a cancer treatment,"[49] while Dr Charles Moertel, who led the Mayo Clinic part of the trial, concluded Laetrile was "ineffective."[50] He reported that 50 percent of patients demonstrated evidence of cancer progression, 90 percent progressed after three months, and 50 percent died before five months. While 19 percent showed improvement in how they felt during the study, the authors attributed this to the placebo effect.[51] The results were resoundingly critical. As he put it, "People have said that crocodile dung and leeching have helped to cure disease based on anecdotal evidence. It is destructive information. We need scientific evidence and now we have it with Laetrile."[52]

Patient-consumer groups reacted very differently to the news. Despite the unfavourable results, in both philosophical and practical terms groups such as the International Association of Cancer Victims and Friends, the Committee for Freedom of Choice in Cancer Therapy, and American Biologics Inc. continued to support the availability and use of Laetrile for cancer. Their rights as patient-consumers, they argued, were being violated; more specifically, they levelled criticisms at the NCI trials. For example, Robert Bradford, founder of the Committee for Freedom of Choice, stated unequivocally that the entire episode was an effort to discredit Laetrile. In his estimation, the NCI "sabotaged the trials to save face" and the negative results meant "nothing."[53] Michael Culbert, editor of Choice, believed genuine Laetrile was never used during the trials. Both Bradford and Culbert launched three separate lawsuits against the NCI, but all three were subsequently dismissed. By contrast, other health interest groups, including the Health Research Group, were critical of the government's response to Laetrile supporters. The NCI's tests, according to Dr Sidney Wolfe, set "an unfortunate precedent" and, at a cost of $400,000–$500,000, were "a waste of money." While the trials may have helped create consensus on Laetrile's effectiveness, Wolfe argued, "patients might have benefited from other experimental drugs."[54] Quackery, according to his logic, was provided a public forum by the NCI.

In 1978, the iconic film actor Steve McQueen developed a cough; he couldn't get rid of it. A year later he had trouble breathing. Famous for *Bullitt*, *The Great Escape*, and *The Thomas Crown Affair*, among others, McQueen was regarded in popular culture as the "King of Cool," a nonconforming underdog, and a racecar-driving rebel. By December of 1979, physicians diagnosed him with mesothelioma, an incurable form of cancer which lined the lungs and was often related to asbestos exposure. In Marc Eliot's penetrating biography, he recounts how McQueen, who had struggled in tumultuous relationships, and with drugs and alcohol, kept the cancer secret from the public. His story went public in March 1980, when *The National Enquirer* ran an article chronicling his "heroic battle against terminal cancer," even though McQueen had desperately sought to appear healthful, even virile. He had recently married Barbara Minty in January and signed on to do another movie called *The Hunter*.[55] He also sent his lawyers after the *Enquirer* to quell speculation. Attorney Ken Ziffren, for example, told the press that "a bronchial ailment" was the reason behind McQueen's hospital stay and the reportage was "untrue, damaging, and actionable."[56] When confronted about his illness, the bad boy actor called it "a bunch of shit." Why McQueen was so bent on repudiating stories of his sickness can only be speculated on, but after ineffective radiotherapy and chemotherapy treatments at Cedars-Sinai Medical Center in Beverly Hills, he was forced to seek alternatives. He had only months to live.

Always an outsider and ever the rebel, McQueen now found himself on the fringes of mainstream cancer therapy. He soon embarked on a journey into the underground medical marketplace and became, much like Ron Woodroof in *Dallas Buyers Club*, a medical tourist. Testifying to the "fear and anxiety" of those desperately ill, McQueen was brutally honest. "When you're in my shoes, you'll grab at anything that's been known to work." Some of the alternatives to orthodox cancer care included homeopathy, such as vitamin and mineral injections. According to his new wife,

"If Steve believed in something, he wasn't going to let the fact that it was not approved by the government stop him."[57] However, the actor did not become a medical tourist eagerly, and his faith in Laetrile followed the exhaustion of all other *American* options.[58] In April, McQueen met with an unscrupulous shady physician named Dr Kelley, who had had his dental licence revoked, been barred from the American Cancer Society, and been investigated by the Internal Revenue Service, among other government agencies. Kelley had recently opened a private – and expensive – health clinic in Rosarito, Mexico, and convinced McQueen to visit. They hit it off, according to Barbara. Normally Steve found physicians uptight, but Kelley was different. He was more down-to-earth and laid back. In August, with no other options, Steve travelled to Kelley's recently opened facility in Mexico. While there, he "received not only pancreatic enzymes but 50 daily vitamins and minerals, massages, prayer sessions, psychotherapy, coffee enemas and injections of a cell preparation made from sheep and cattle fetuses."[59] He was given chiropractic treatments, massages, daily sauna sessions, and marujama (not marijuana), a Japanese extract of tuberculosis bacilli Z. Finally, McQueen was placed on a diet that included only organically grown fruit and vegetables and raw certified milk, in addition to Laetrile.

Remarkably, he began to improve, but only for a short while. With the disease having metastasized to his abdomen, chest, and back, his bounce-back was near-miraculous. When the media tracked him down in October, he made statements of the Mexican government's willingness to allow him a degree of therapeutic autonomy. "Mexico," he said, "is showing the world a new way of fighting cancer through nonspecific metabolic therapies."[60] *People* magazine ran a feature in its October issue and cast a spotlight on Kelley, as well as his business partner, Dr Rodrigo Rodriguez. According to the latter, the clinic's program was meant to "build up the immune system" and individual treatments were calculated by computer after the submission of a 2,500-item questionnaire. McQueen also thanked his fans in a message that was broadcast across the globe. The American medical establishment dismissed Kelley's clinical practice as charlatanism and McQueen's message of medical freedom, yet the dying actor certainly raised public awareness of Laetrile. Many wanted to hear about his ostensible recovery. Many wanted to know about the viability of this contested medicine.

In November 1980 – just a month later – McQueen died after surgery to remove cancerous masses. He had briefly provided many cancer-stricken Americans and their families a rallying point and beacon of hope, something that would resonate after his passing. Media reported that "McQueen's experience in Mexico pursuing the alternative cancer treatment spawned an exodus of thousands with terminal cancer to seek similar treatments in Mexico following his death."[61] Historian Barron Lerner argued in his book *When Illness Goes Public* that McQueen fostered the growth of complementary medicine in the US more generally. His ashes were scattered in the Pacific Ocean. Four days after his death, the *Star* reported how "Desperate Cancer Patients Are Flocking to Mexico Seeking Steve McQueen's Therapy."[62]

CONCLUSION

Pro-Laetrile groups were antagonized by the federal government's approach to Laetrile and regarded the decision to oppose its use as emblematic of a broadly intrusive and imperious government. Even though there was no substantive proof underpinning Laetrile's claim of effectiveness, its proponents still sought to legalize it. Advocates for Laetrile, including Bradford, Culbert, and Symms, argued that sick Americans had the freedom to choose any therapy they wanted – be it in the United States, Mexico, or Morocco. These advocates lobbied politicians hard to this end. Representatives in the House, responding to their constituents, introduced bills that would have legalized Laetrile, but they subsequently failed to generate the requisite votes. Similarly, Laetrile's supporters challenged the constitutionality of the 1962 effectiveness requirement on the basis of personal freedom. Lawyers contended during proceedings that the Kefauver efficacy amendment should not apply to drugs for persons with a fatal illness for which there was no conventional cure, even if the evidence in support of that drug was anecdotal; ultimately this line of reasoning was unsuccessful. The Food and Drug Administration, for its part, fought against pro-Laetrile advocates vigorously.[63]

Amid an ongoing war on cancer and the war on drugs, the Laetrile episode underscored valuable lessons that would have great import during future debates over legitimate medicines. More than that, Laetrile provided object lessons in how to deal with medical constituencies, including during the AIDS epidemic in the 1980s. Indeed,

Laetrile was a forerunner of events in the 1980s, when individuals such as Lewis Engman, head of the Pharmaceutical Manufacturers Association, enunciated a faith in the sanctity of free choice, personal freedom, and the patient's right to choose a medication. The Laetrile debate centred on the same fundamental principle: free choice in the marketplace. First, the dispute over Laetrile brought into sharp focus the need for the FDA's managerial staff, its key decision-makers, to recognize the influence of a persistent freedom-of-choice argument in a landscape of doubt and fear. Government appointees, career employees in health, and elected officials had to ask themselves hard questions about the price of business-as-usual versus institutional flexibility in the face of widespread public pressure. Should average Americans, whether terminal cancer patients or AIDS patients, be permitted to spend their money any way they wanted? On any drug they wanted, however spurious, however hazardous? At what stage should such persons be allowed access to experimental, yet unapproved, drugs?

Second, in the wake of the Laetrile episode, the FDA – more specifically – gleaned that it was vital to safeguard its use of the scientific method and normal regulatory standard practices, and thereby shield patients from ineffective drugs. To this end, the FDA aggressively shored up regulatory requirements and standards, as it instituted new benchmarks aimed at better protecting the nation's drug supply. Called good clinical practices (GCPs), the requirements included: informed consent of participants in a clinical trial, ethical evaluation by local institutional review boards, monitoring of clinical studies for adherence to protocol and data integrity, timely reporting of adverse events, and periodic reports to the FDA.

The Laetrile experience aroused key public policy questions concerning the roles of medicine and science, of regulatory and research agencies, of lawmakers and courts of law, and of the drug regulatory system embodied in the Federal Food, Drug, and Cosmetic Act and carried out by the Food and Drug Administration.[64] These questions went unanswered. Instead, the debate over Laetrile epitomized the growing complexity of the FDA's task in establishing the correct equilibrium between consumer protection, innovation, and access. A potent Laetrile movement encouraged cancer patients to feel that, by using Laetrile, they were not only availing themselves of a safe and effective remedy, but also somehow collaborating in an effort to "show up" the orthodox medical establishment. This, in turn, forced the FDA to describe its institutional identity to both regulatory reformers and consumer activists.

Proponents of Laetrile continue to push back against the encroachment of the FDA. Dr Josh Axe, who has appeared on *The Dr. Oz Show*, recommends the use of vitamin B-17 (Laetrile) as a supplementary cancer treatment, but contends that "most agree it shouldn't be the primary cancer treatment for any patient." Nor is it "approved for cancer prevention or cancer use in the United States." This is because "the FDA feels that more information is needed regarding the effects of vitamin B17 in human clinical trials before it can be widely used." As such, his website suggests it ought to be taken in as natural a form as possible to sidestep the side effects of a potent concentration, while simultaneously pointing out that Laetrile can still be obtained "from Mexico, where vitamin B17 production for medicinal purpose[s] is still supported." Laughably, the recommendation also indicates that "it's not illegal to possess or use."[65] Dr Axe has no medical training, and does not possess a licence to practise as a physician. As a "certified doctor of natural medicine" who believes in "using food as medicine," he practises naturopathy.[66] Using the language of "feeling" in lieu of evidence-based information, he offers patient-consumers an "alternative" set of facts to make their own minds up about vitamin B-17 (Laetrile). Perhaps it should not be surprising, but decades after the Laetrile controversy there are still those who urge sick individuals to follow Steve McQueen's trek to Mexico for unapproved cancer treatment.

In increasing numbers, Americans have begun travelling to Mexico for a range of medical procedures, not just for Laetrile or HIV/AIDS drugs. The border towns of Tijuana and Mexicali, for instance, offer tummy tucks, facelifts, and dental surgeries for a fraction of what such treatments cost at home. Moreover, towns on the northern US border have become destinations for Canadians unwilling to wait months for a doctor's appointment in their own country. Globalization and advances in technology, in short, have transformed the nature of health care, making procedures such as remote diagnoses and telesurgery – in which a surgeon can operate on a distant patient by using a robotically controlled arm – a more common practice. Lastly, cheaper travel has led to increasing numbers of people crossing the globe for medical care.

Part Two

HIPPY MEDICINE

4

LSD'S RETURN FROM THE WILDERNESS

In 2015, the *British Medical Journal* challenged its readers to rethink the therapeutic potential of certain psychedelic drugs. The *BMJ* was not alone in issuing such a call. *Scientific American* had produced an editorial column the year before calling for an end to the ban on psychedelic drug research. *The Lancet* did much the same. In arguing that the demonization of psychedelic drugs as a "social evil" bottled up critical medical research, the world's leading medical journals were collectively lamenting the sacrifice of a superior understanding of the brain and better treatments for conditions such as depression.[1] The articles, in different ways, criticized the mental health authorities for failing to advance therapies beyond the golden era of the 1950s, and lambasted drug regulators for prohibiting psychedelic drugs, including LSD, Ecstasy (MDMA), and psilocybin: drugs which had historically held clinical promise but were "designated as drugs of abuse."[2] Some prominent psychiatrists, including Ben Sessa, said the field was static. "We all in psychiatry know we need innovation. Because we are stuck and we know it. Our treatment outcomes are not that much better than they were 75 years ago." As Sessa argued, psychedelic medicines represented an advancement that ought to be embraced.[3]

Older drugs (lithium in 1949, chlorpromazin in 1952, imipramin in 1957, haloperidol in 1958, and diazepam in 1963) changed the face of psychiatry and quickly became major pillars of psychiatric treatment. Historian Edward Shorter has characterized the period as the beginning of "the second biological psychiatry," whereas psychopharmacologist David Healy pronounced that a "therapeutic revolution" was the immediate outcome of the 1950s–60s. The editors of *Scientific American* pointed out that the situation created a classic Catch-22 that would make Captain John Yossarian proud. The outsider drugs were "banned because they have no accepted medical use, but researchers cannot explore their therapeutic potential because they are banned."[4] According to Sessa, "the psychiatric community are kind of ready to grasp psychedelics." This was the case, he added, because "[p]sychiatrists, like other doctors, they just want safe and efficacious treatments for their patients. If it works and it's safe, they will use it."[5] Pieces in *The New Yorker*, *The Atlantic*, and other major periodicals followed on the heels of the BMJ, *Scientific American*, and *The Lancet*, and they discussed the relative safety and efficacy of LSD. Altogether, these periodicals brought attention to a growing contention amongst researchers, and even some regulators, that a moral panic about drug abuse – rather than a more rational approach based on scientific evidence – stymied the clinical potential of psychedelic drugs.[6] These publications signalled that perhaps LSD was returning from the wilderness.

In this chapter, I examine the career of LSD from its earliest trials to contemporary debates in the twenty-first century. This work builds upon the findings of historian Erika Dyck as well as anthropologist Nicolas Langlitz, whose careful study of LSD in neuroscience has provided the groundwork for examining the contemporary science of psychedelics.[7] His description of the laboratory research of both Franz Vollenweider and Mark Geyer, for instance, draws attention to how scientists have altered their research approaches in response to regulations relevant to not only LSD, but also Ecstasy and ketamine, and the other drugs in this book. According to British psychopharmacologist David Nutt, LSD, among other psychoactive drugs, has viable therapeutic applications, yet existing restrictions in both laboratories and clinical trials have prevented exploration of its therapeutic potential due to long-standing notions of harm. In 1967, the "snowball was set on its way" and "there was little hard information about this curious substance." A decade later, in 1977, Ralph Metzner reported that LSD was in a "holding pattern, waiting for the general change in consciousness to occur."[8] Metzner, like Nutt and the editors of *Scientific American*, has lamented the holding pattern, and in particular the "daunting bureaucratic labyrinth" that dissuades "even the most committed investigator."[9]

THE UPS AND COME-DOWNS OF LSD

In 1938, Albert Hofmann, a Swiss biochemist working at Sandoz Pharmaceutical Laboratories, synthesized Lysergic acid-diethylamide-25, an internal name applied to the twenty-fifth compound in the lysergic acid series.[10] On Friday 16 April 1943, Hofmann had his first LSD experience, though he had not realized that he had come into contact with the chemical and the response stupefied him. During the phase of disorientation, he "perceived an uninterrupted stream of fantastic pictures, extraordinary shapes and an intense, kaleidoscopic play of colors."[11] In LSD: *My Problem Child*, he famously reflected on the drug that he discovered in an honest and incisive manner. The book captured the maddening mixture of excitement and joy he experienced with the new discovery and his high – pardon the pun – hopes for this chemical.[12]

Thereafter, Sandoz Pharmaceuticals began experiments with LSD, first in animal models, and ultimately within the field of psychiatry. The drug's effects attracted researchers working in mental health. Some, in particular, found it useful due to its rather consistent capacity to affect cognition and induce a period of reflection among users.[13] LSD quickly gripped the minds of clinical, bio-medical, spiritual, and political thinkers traversing the disciplinary spectrum. Its unconventional status, too, meant that it rapidly became divisive. By the early 1960s, over a thousand scientific articles had appeared with investigators using LSD in a wide variety of settings, applying diverse methods and instruments, and drawing a number of different conclusions. Glin Bennet wrote in the *BJP* that some 1,500 studies would be shelved.[14] According to Michael Pollan, "between 1953 and 1973, the federal government spent four million dollars to fund a hundred and sixteen studies of LSD, involving more than seventeen hundred subjects. (These figures do not include classified research.) Through the mid-nineteen-sixties, psilocybin and LSD were legal and remarkably easy to obtain."[15] By no means did the research community reach consensus on a precise direction for LSD studies, but a number of promising avenues emerged throughout the 1950s. Principal among these was the use of LSD for treating alcoholism; then again, it was also tested in clinical settings on a range of behaviours, including homosexuality, depression, and aggression, for couples therapy, and as a model psychosis.[16]

While researchers subscribed to diverse methods for testing LSD, its appeal broadened to include non-clinical investigations and the drug was heralded as a vehicle for spiritual and creative thoughts.[17] Individuals tried to harness these reactions and put them to productive use in clinical settings, even as others recognized the desire to move beyond the confines of medicine and perhaps better serve us by enriching human thinking along evolutionary terms. Some of those thinkers acknowledged a longer tradition of hallucinogens that connected with traditional healing practices among Aboriginal people or linked them with non-traditional religions.[18] North American investigators looked to the use of peyote among members of the Native American Church, for instance, a religious organization that had steadily spread northward from Mexico in the twentieth century. Exploring religious interactions with hallucinogenic substances encouraged scientists to consider how spiritual and psychological healing had been historically one and the same.[19] Others looked to ololiuqui use among the Aztecs, who similarly derived meaning from drug-induced visions or hallucinations.[20]

In 1957, psychiatrist Humphry Osmond, then working in a mental hospital in Saskatchewan, coined the term "psychedelic," which was a nod to the substance's mind-manifesting properties and a description of how the drug brought psychological material to light.[21] Although Osmond derived the name through his correspondence with American writer Aldous Huxley, famous for *Brave New World*, its meaning was connected to his clinical work with alcoholics alongside his theory that LSD produced a model psychosis that provided insights into schizophrenia. He, along with his colleagues in Saskatchewan, believed that LSD, along with other psychedelic drugs, including peyote (mescaline), ololiuqui, and others, provided western medicine with a critical tool for linking biomedical approaches with spiritual and psychological healing – a feature that had been leached away by modern medical interventions that tended to favour body over spirit. Even more, he felt strongly that such drugs could aid in the understanding as well as the treatment of schizophrenia and other disorders.[22] Following World War II, Osmond took up a position at the psychiatric unit at St George's Hospital, in London. There, he and Dr John Smythies embarked on collaborative research into chemically induced reactions in the body. Mescaline, in particular, drew the attention of Osmond and Smythies; and after testing the peyote-extracted hallucinogen on volunteers, they realized its effects on patients were "similar to people's experience of schizophrenia."[23]

These findings had major repercussions for their partnership. They not only developed a theory that schizophrenia stemmed from a biochemical imbalance in the sufferer, but Osmond and Smythies further criticized what they deemed old-fashioned treatment methods for the disorder. These methods included insulin, water, electricity, or psychosocial therapy, among others. With insulin shock therapy, doctors would inject insulin into psychotic, drug-addicted, or schizophrenic patients, thereby causing them to become hypoglycemic and go into comas.[24] Water therapy, by contrast, also known as "pro-baths," involved the use of water and wet packs to assuage a patient's agitation. According to a more sinister account of the practice, this therapy sometimes meant a patient was strapped into a canvas bag in a large bathtub then subjected to both cold and hot water. In this rendering, it was a "medieval form of shock therapy."[25] In the early years of electroconvulsive shock therapy, patients were given unmodified treatments (straight ECT), which meant they were not given any muscle relaxants or anesthetic. On rare occasions, this caused fractures or dislocations of long bones.[26] Last, the psychosocial approach emphasized such remedies as cognitive behavioural therapy, community treatment, family treatment, and various other treatments.

Believing they knew better, Osmond and Smythies created a grandiose research program aimed at understanding both the psychological and biochemical nature of schizophrenia. This double blow at the established norms surrounding schizophrenia resulted in frosty working relations at the hospital. As Osmond grew increasingly aware that his colleagues, mainly psychoanalysts, were indifferent or even hostile to such a biochemical investigation, he decided to pursue his work elsewhere.[27] In October 1951, Osmond uprooted himself from his native England and emigrated to Weyburn, Saskatchewan, where his ideas about schizophrenia could be nurtured. He arrived at a propitious moment: a new provincial government, led by T.C. Douglas, had recently initiated a profound medical transformation, an experiment in socialized medicine that would eventually influence the rest of Canada.[28]

Apart from schizophrenia, LSD's use in treating alcoholism gathered significant attention throughout the 1950s, even within more conventional treatment modalities. The therapeutic approach involved single doses, albeit mega-doses, of LSD. Patients were required to sit with a counselor (sometimes a psychologist, psychiatrist, nurse, or social worker), usually for an entire day. Patients were encouraged to talk about themselves, often prompted by looking at family photographs or while listening to classical music, or by looking at artwork. Results after follow-up studies indicated a high degree of sobriety following these sessions. Individuals, likewise, claimed that they had generated a new level of self-awareness and psychological fortitude to end their drinking problem.[29] The results thwarted contemporary addictions researchers, some of whom were less comfortable with a drug trial that did not conform to the emerging standards of randomized controlled testing.[30]

These promising avenues of research, in part, helped convince regulators that LSD was worth pursuing as a clinical substance. Besides, during the 1950s, as David Healy has shown, these drugs were among hundreds of new substances flooding the market during the golden age of psychopharmacology.[31] Prior to the 1950s, Healy explains, drug research existed in a dark age – that is, before the advent of the anti-psychotic chlorpromazine, which ushered in the modern era of psychopharmacotherapy.[32] Within this decade of pharmaceutical confidence and expansion, LSD entered the scene as one among many substances competing for clinical attention. In spite of its now notorious qualities, immense potential characterized its early years. The next phase of its life demonstrated that it had a wilder side.

TURBULENT TIMES AND RADICAL PSYCHIATRY

By the beginning of the 1960s LSD had become a familiar substance within bio-medical research circles, but it had yet to reach ordinary society in any meaningful way. Ken Kesey was then a creative writing student at Stanford University who had volunteered to take LSD as part of a clinical trial before he leapt onto the psychedelic scene as a champion of LSD-induced mind freedom.[33] Timothy Leary had explored a variety of drugs – both personally and professionally – before landing in trouble with Harvard University for his "unscientific" use of psilocybin mushrooms and drug experiments with prison inmates.[34]

These two figures became connected with a different side of LSD's character by the mid-1960s. During that contested decade, LSD's reputation changed significantly. Leary catapulted from Harvard University to Millbrook, an elite upstate New York getaway for acid jamborees, where he established himself as a spiritual leader and principal interpreter of the psychedelic gospel. "In each generation," according to Leary's promotional literature, "a few men stumble upon the riddle of consciousness and its solutions."[35] He was one such man. Ken Kesey, meanwhile, had published his exposé of American mental hospitals in *One Flew Over the Cuckoo's Nest* and was quickly coupled with a rising tide of countercultural shenanigans, which included his rather flamboyant consumption of drugs.[36] Throughout North America, psychedelics coursed through 1960s culture, inciting new genres of music, literature, hedonism, and anti-authority attitudes. While many of these relationships were exaggerated, the presumed connection between LSD and immorality overwhelmed a more rational assessment of the situation.[37]

Along with Leary, for example, a fellow psychologist, Arthur Kleps, promoted a mixture of mysticism and reformism that he hoped might fundamentally alter the trajectory of the United States. He was optimistic, too, that he would cure the country – not just the individual – with LSD, love, and increased awareness of the self. For gurus such as Kleps, in short, it was not just about hedonism. As a means to understand the inner self, LSD was a pathway to casting off individual neuroses. But it was also a tool for national redemption and rejuvenation. Together, Leary, Brotherhood members, and Kleps sought to challenge the status quo and rectify long-standing psychoses in society through LSD spirituality. And if radicals in the psy-sciences had Laing's *Divided Self* and Szasz's *Myth of Mental Illness* as guides to define their ideas and actions, then Leary's *The Psychedelic Experience: A Manual Based on the Tibetan Book of the Dead* and Kleps's *The Boo Hoo Bible: The Neo-American Church Catechism and Handbook* served as similar handbooks.

Another so-called radical was R.D. Laing, who also employed LSD as part of his therapeutic armamentarium. Born in the Govanhill district of Glasgow on 7 October 1927, the only child of David Park MacNair Laing and Amelia Glen Laing, young Ronald Laing was clever, competitive, and talented.[38] He thoroughly enjoyed reading Classics, particularly philosophy, and was a gifted musician, and was eventually made an Associate of the Royal College of Music. Still, he chose to go on to study medicine at the University of Glasgow. He conducted radical institutional experiments while stationed at Gartnavel Royal Hospital, and then at the private community clinic of Kingsley Hall. Laing's books regularly topped bestseller lists in the US; he shared the same stage as such iconic bands as the Grateful Dead, acted as a guru to the Beatles, was featured in *Life* and *Esquire* (as well as lesser-known, more avant-garde publications such as *Oz* or *The New Internationalist*), and was often the centre of commotion, positive *and* negative. The psychiatric establishment regularly tried to close his community at Kingsley Hall, for instance, seeing his occasional therapeutic use of LSD and his belief in meta-noia (self-healing) as simultaneously irresponsible and unscientific.[39]

Laing, in short, became something of a celebrity doctor him-self, and even if he was working on the borders of orthodox men-tal health practice, he was not alone. In discussing teaching at the Castalia Foundation and Tim Leary's Millbrook Institute, Laing noted that medical practitioners were using LSD across the UK, in places such as the Clinical Theology Centre, Nottingham; the Shenley Mental Hospital; and the Institute of Mental Imagery, in Cambridge.[40] He knew that another Ronald – Ronald Sandison – was using LSD in Scotland. And he was knowledgeable about the clinical use of LSD (and other substances such as mescalin) in places such as Saskatchewan and Hollywood Hospital, British Columbia. As for its curative power and perceived and real dangers, he was keenly aware that LSD was "the subject of considerable controversy both inside and outside professional journals."[41] In peer-reviewing a colleague's work on the substance, Laing argued that "LSD appears to be neither a drug of addiction nor a drug of habituation. I agree of course that it should not be employed irresponsibly."[42] Indeed, he used it in regular practice, and to treat a range of mental health problems, ranging from schizophrenia to heroin addiction.

Apart from Laing, radical psychiatry's criticism of mainstream psy-chiatry's role in Vietnam and militarism connected tangentially to LSD and other drugs such as cannabis. Many mental health figures rebelled against the use of psychological adjustment or the weaponization of psychiatry in any form: mind control, LSD brainwashing. Even more anodyne procedures such as therapy for soldiers were critiqued. So, when it was revealed that the Bureau of Narcotics was involved in highly classified psychological research, various radical psychiatrists and anti-psychiatrists reacted with a mixture of fury and forbearance. Harry J. Anslinger himself conducted experimental research with nar-cotics that focused on ways to control human behaviour and break down psychological defences in enemy agents. "We are trying to dis-cover a truth drug," Anslinger admitted in 1968, "by using peyote and sodium amytal." They also resorted to marijuana, which he had called the "killer weed."*[43] At the American Orthopsychiatric Association annual meeting in 1970, Paul Lowinger noted, "health professionals have a responsibility to speak to the public on issues which involve freedom, health, and human behavior." Besides issues of access to services and more comprehensive health care for the general public, he was specifically referring to the "voluminous rhetoric" around such drugs as marijuana, amphetamines, and LSD, which had become "emotionally charged issues."[44]

Lowinger, who was one of the founders of the Radical Caucus in the American Psychiatric Association, was also a prolific researcher and writer. He was an organizer and advocate. Along with other self-proclaimed radical psychiatrists, Lowinger helped to strengthen, if not completely clarify, the position of his peers. Over his career, he wrote on eclectic but unsurprising topics, including doctors as political activists, LSD, marijuana, psychosurgery, prison reform, and, not surprisingly, the features of radical psychiatry, although he focused on grander "social forces of progress" and what he perceived as "independence of thought and action" that underpinned much of his work.[45] Unlike many of his counterparts, throughout his career he largely avoided talk of violent revolution and tearing down existing structures. Striking a middle-ground approach, Lowinger proclaimed in 1967 during a wide-ranging Conference on Radicals in the Professions that his fellow psychiatrists "need not be reactionary, conservative or passive in the face of revolutionary social change."[46]

In the popular press, LSD was associated with murder, suicide, and a chain of health problems, alongside a more generalized set of antipathies towards the American state.[47] High on acid and caught in terrifying hallucinations, it was thought that young people might be driven to madness and bloodshed. Charles Manson's serial murders were attributed to LSD; elsewhere a former medical student reportedly murdered his mother; LSD-soaked youths contracted venereal diseases at concerts; others went blind after taking LSD and believing they could stare at the sun.[48] Within the realm of cinema, Jack Nicholson proved crucial in interpreting and promoting both anti-establishment concepts and psychedelic iconography in film. In *The*

* Physicians also used to give sodium amytal to soldiers in the US Army in World War II when they were conducting "abreaction" therapy for battle exhaustion (combat stress/ trauma).

Trip (1967), *Psych-Out* (1968), and *Easy Rider* (1969), Nicholson contributed as both actor and writer to the loosely structured sub-genre known as the psychedelic film or "head movie." Having low budgets with overlapping actors (Dennis Hopper, Henry Fonda, Bruce Dern, Susan Strasberg), the three Nicholson films employed creative, trippy qualities, including "abstract color patterns, disjunctive editing, gratuitous excesses of camera placement and movement, and extreme lens effects."[49] Furthermore, the experimental and often non-linear format was designed to make the film experience a transforming and pleasurable experience for the viewer, even if the plot was far from straightforward or satisfying. Nicholson and director Roger Corman, with whom he was working, did not pioneer the genre alone, since *The Love Statue: LSD Experience* (1965), *LSD, I Hate You* (1966), *Hallucination Generation* (1966), and *The Love-Ins* (1967) were all released earlier, or at least contemporaneously. Nicholson, for his part, never explicitly acknowledged his desire to push the trend, nor were the films particularly successful, with the exception of *Easy Rider*, which was both critically acclaimed and a countercultural touchstone. Released in 1969, it was foreshadowed by a *New York Times* article a year earlier that underlined the growth of the psychedelic film genre, where it was pronounced that "there should be little doubt at this stage the moviemakers are involved in the world of LSD."[50]

While sociologists have since identified that the madness-inducing claims about LSD were hyperbolic, medical researchers found themselves snared in a moral panic over the value of LSD. Sandoz, undeniably worried about its reputation, temporarily suspended production of its LSD supplies in 1963. It became plain that other substances had seeped onto the black market masquerading as LSD when in fact they bore no chemical similarities.[51] The rise of drug use in general, and psychedelics in particular, created challenges for medical researchers faced with the growing reputation that these substances were merely agents of abuse. In a similar way, medical staff had trouble handling patients who claimed to have taken LSD, when the drugs in circulation were often not bona fide LSD, and were often consumed in combination with other substances that further confused staff attempting to manage a drug reaction or presumed overdose.

As public concerns heightened over the dangers associated with LSD use, drug regulators at first worked closely with scientists to determine how best to regulate this drug. In the early 1960s, clinical optimism had tipped the scales in favour of a regulatory scheme that allowed for continued investigations along rather liberal lines. Some researchers maintained that LSD was on the cusp of making significant breakthroughs in addiction treatment and that further sustained study was necessary to see through the haze of misinformation surrounding the recreational abuse of the drug. Then, the Kefauver Harris Drug Amendments (1962) introduced more stringent requirements for proving a drug's efficacy, and this pushed researchers to focus on trial design over therapeutic method. The novel nature of LSD therapy complicated how scientists pigeonholed their data within the new regulatory framework, marking the beginning of the end of LSD clinical research.[52]

Elsewhere, acid on the streets wreaked havoc and induced psychotic breakdowns in otherwise sane people, according to news, police, and health reports. Bellevue Hospital in New York City stated that it had never before received so many patients into its psychiatric division, but had admitted 65 people in 1965 alone with LSD-induced psychoses. Fully nine of those cases involved "uncontrolled violent urges including homicide attempts by 2 individuals. Four others were found running or sitting nude in the streets."[53] The states of New York and California convened Senate hearings in 1966 to outlaw LSD. The Canadian government had responded four years earlier with a more tepid response, placing LSD alongside thalidomide on a special new drug schedule reserved for drugs that were still under medical investigation, but which were not otherwise controlled through the criminal justice system. Leaders of the psychedelic movement, including psychologist Timothy Leary, writer Ken Kesey, poet Allen Ginsberg, and others, had become the new face of the drug and spoke fluently about the conservatism of the state in attempting to stamp out a form of cultural consciousness. These self-declared defenders of psychedelia forged a robust popular connection between LSD and counter-culture hedonism that may have galvanized supporters, but also certainly severed them off from mainstream society. The resulting cultural division cut deeply across conventional authority figures, including psychedelic researchers, who risked being labelled as unethical scientists or unpatriotic citizens by association.

In 1968, pressure came from all directions to regulate LSD out of legal territory completely. The scientific community could not come to an agreement on whether LSD's potential might actually be realized. While some researchers balked at its inability to perform consistently in controlled trials, others chided the spiritual dimension assigned to its healing potential. Either way, it had not sufficiently insinuated itself into a specific disease category or sought-after psychopharmaceutical position to warrant further evaluation. Volunteers for trials also gradually came from a less desirable segment of society – those seeking thrills, rather than legitimate, or even objective, test subjects. The capacity of researchers to establish quantifiable and verifiable results thus became ever more challenging.[54] Politically, it became increasingly demanding to justify further studies of LSD while it appeared to produce violent and sustained health problems, primarily within psychiatric categories. Results, whether in clinical trials or on the streets, seemed to produce startlingly unpredictable and highly dangerous outcomes, leaving politicians and regulators no choice but to step in and restore public confidence in their ability to decrease public health risks.

By the 1970s, the psychedelic arena was considerably dissimilar to what it had been in the 1950s. Funded, legitimate scientific research directly using LSD largely stopped, while committed enthusiasts continued to manufacture the drug illegally and fuel an underground network of research. Recreationally, LSD continued to be a force and was now swiftly joined by a mass of other narcotics: psychedelics from peyote to mushrooms, and other substances from the relatively benign marijuana, to a range of contraband pills of speed, to injectable heroin. The drug cornucopia, which had always been present but highly regulated, exploded onto the scene with renewed eagerness as it commingled with ideas about consciousness-raising philosophies, anti-authoritarian attitudes, and risk-averse liberties. The term "psychedelic" was invested with new meanings. Lisa Bieberman, for example, who had been with Leary at the founding of his movement, came out against him. For her, the movement now represented "gaudy illegible posters, gaudy unreadable tabloids, loud parties and anything paisley, crowded noisy discotheques, trinket shops and the slum districts that patronize them."[55]

Not without some irony, this was also the era of psychopharmacology, when more pharmaceuticals moved into circulation than ever before. These drug scenes also disproportionately involved middle-class America. Regulators drew a sharp line between approved middle-class pharmaceutical consumption, such as Valium or Miltown, and middle-class drug abuse, including LSD. The tone of psychedelic research shifted from studies within the realm of pharmaceutical trials to ones exploring spiritual, philosophical, and cultural dimensions of the relationship between reality and consciousness. These kinds of questions moved beyond the comfort zone of modern western medicine and developed small enclaves outside of university campuses.[56] As Bieberman argued in the pages of the *New Republic*:

> A tool of tremendous potential value for science, medicine and personal life enrichment has been allowed, partly by default, to become the plaything of unscrupulous cultists ... Whether one places the blame for its corruption on the politicians who drove LSD underground, on the academicians who allowed this to happen, or on the opportunists who took advantage of the result, the fact remains that society could hardly have done a more thorough job of confounding the good, and magnifying the evil potential in these powerful drugs if that had been the avowed intention of all concerned.[57]

LSD research moved underground while its more social persona took on a life of its own, leaching into cultural products, music, literature, and the visual arts as it became intertwined into the fabric of the 1960s, making appearances only in times of desperation, whether in emergency rooms or in jail cells.[58] This phase of LSD's career seemed extreme enough to overwhelm any future consideration of its use for valid medical therapies.

"TABOO" AND COMEBACK

Not so. In recent years, LSD has emerged from its reclusive existence and, alongside other psychedelics such as methylenedioxy-N-methylamphethamine (MDMA, aka Ecstasy) and psilocybin (magic mushrooms), is now the subject of well-funded and well-regulated basic research in Great Britain, the United States, and Switzerland. A "medical research taboo" no more, LSD-25 is being examined as a potential treatment in alcoholism, post-traumatic stress disorder, and cluster headaches, and as an adjunct in palliative care; in the field of neuroscience, it is being investigated for its ability to reveal brain functions and provide a more sophisticated grasp of cognition.[59] Finally, a third approach is how it creates or influences mystical/religious experiences. For Andrew Brown, writing in *The Spectator*, this "psychedelic revival" in scientific and medical research is far removed from the "wackier end of the pro-LSD lobby."[60] Yet, for all the progress that LSD has made in the past decade, there have been no major breakthroughs, no marketable prescription drugs, and division continues to characterize the scientific community and regulatory authorities. The drug's career cycle has certainly entered a new phase, one of contentiousness and upheaval. It continues to be haunted by its checkered past while regulators and politicians are reluctant to loosen the grip on psychedelics, affecting the way that researchers design their studies. One wonders if this might pass with another generation, as LSD and the 1960s connection fade in people's memory and the last living people who remember the 60s are gone. As one psychiatrist put it recently, "the psychedelic 1960s is a bit of a misnomer," because "this is the psychedelic era."[61]

In this latest rejuvenation of LSD research, various actors and organizations have driven the career cycle and, more particularly, its revival as an object of study. Champions, including the Beckley Foundation, the Council of Spiritual Practices, the Heffter Research Institute, and the Multidisciplinary Association for Psychedelic Studies (MAPS), among others, have formed a network that offers institutional support and financial resources to sustain studies. These groups have survived in part by embracing the technocratic and bureaucratic elements of drug development and keeping the countercultural baggage of the earlier psychedelic movement at arm's length. Among these, none have been more instrumental than MAPS, which began originally as the relaunched non-profit Earth Metabolic Design Lab (EMDL) in the mid-1980s. Indeed, LSD's revival was a product of this era, when anti-drug rhetoric and legislative initiatives featured prominently.[62]

In 1984, Rick Doblin and Debby Harlow, among others, were disappointed with the Drug Enforcement Administration's recent move to criminalize MDMA and sought to offer a coordinated response from the psychedelic psychotherapy community.[63] Part of the nascent "War on Drugs," the DEA's effort eventually classified MDMA as a Schedule 1 drug, meaning it was designated as having no medical use.[64] With EMDL, and later MAPS, which was founded in 1986, the psychedelic community at least had a vehicle to communicate with the criminal justice system, pharmaceutical industry, DEA, Food and Drug Administration (FDA), and National Institutes of Health (NIH).

Doblin, for his part, was instrumental in the (re)creation of the psychedelic research movement. He established MAPS with the express purpose of bringing psychedelic medications to market, training therapists, supporting research that examined the links between neuroscience, spirituality, and creativity, and educating the public about the risks and benefits of psychedelics.[65] A follower of Dr Stanislav Grof and a tireless supporter of mainstream psychedelic therapy, he was deeply influenced by the Holocaust, the nuclear arms race, and the Vietnam War.[66] He believed that dehumanization, denial, projection, and scapegoating were the core psychological factors associated with these conflicts and that they needed to be addressed in order to build a "healthier, sustainable world."[67] In Doblin's estimation, extant mental health therapies were inadequate to relieve these mental traumas on the individual level or produce meaningful changes at the state and global level.[68] To this end, he believed psychedelics were useful in everyday psychotherapy and ought to be developed as FDA-approved prescription drugs.

From 1986 to 1988, MAPS worked alongside university- and hospital-based researchers to develop and submit to the FDA protocols and produce new drug applications for MDMA human research studies. Yet, the re-emergence of MDMA as an object of research was anything but smooth. All of the applications, including single-patient and double-blind controlled trials, were rejected by the FDA, raising criticism of the agency's supposed lack of evidence-based neutrality. Various researchers, for instance, questioned the FDA's Neuropharmacologic Drug Products Division for basing its decisions on "underlying cultural prejudice against medical research with drugs that were criminalized" and ignoring risk/benefit assessments that were generally favourable. According to David Nichols of Purdue University, a cofounder of the Heffter Research Institute, the subsequent advancement of the psychedelic research agenda in the 1990s and 2000s can be partially explained by a "change in FDA personnel" and a newer "generation of regulators."[69]

In the company of others, LSD has fitfully re-emerged after the phase of its career in which scientific research was driven underground, halted, or discredited. This was welcome news to Albert Hofmann, the discoverer of LSD. Before he died at the age of 102 in 2008, he expressed some pleasure that the "problem child" he had spawned was "in the hands of medical doctors again" and being studied in his native Switzerland.[70] According to Peter Gasser, head of the Swiss Medical Society for Psycholytic Therapy and the principal investigator of an LSD anxiety/illness study, Hofmann's final wish had come to pass with this development. As described by Nicolas Langlitz, LSD had matured again, this time "from wonder and shame to inquiry."[71]

A robust Swiss and American partnership heightened the inquiry. In Switzerland, Gasser's LSD investigation, which was approved by the medical and legal authorities in 2007, became the first study to evaluate the drug's therapeutic applications in nearly four decades. At the same time, the FDA received the same application. In 2008, the FDA joined the Swiss government in accepting the protocol. Gasser presented his research findings in April 2013 at the Mind & Medicine Psychedelic Conference in Oakland, California. His paper, "LSD-Assisted Psychotherapy in the Treatment of Anxiety Secondary to Life Threatening Illness," was met not only with a warm reception but with various questions about the positive data and the dying patient's right to select their own drug in the hospice.[72] In essence, physicians and professionals raised salient points about the complexity of controlling and limiting access to a psychoactive drug for those patients with little to lose. It was a debate, too, that was reminiscent of heroin discussions during the 1980s.

While researchers sought a practical application for LSD in the form of assisted psychotherapy, others, including Dr Mark Geyer and another Swiss, Dr Franz Vollenweider, have found an end route to studying more classical questions associated with LSD (spirituality in healing, cognition, model psychosis). In the early 1990s, Geyer, a world-renowned psychopharmacologist and neuroscientist as well as a cofounder of the Heffter Institute, identified a "highly talented" albeit slightly "scrambled" brain researcher in Zurich. Vollenweider possessed a passionate interest in psychedelics as well as sophisticated neuroimaging technologies, and he operated in a "more permissive drug policy and regulatory regime."[73] He was an intriguing collaborator for Geyer and David Nichols, and became an important ally.

Together, they have initiated research demonstrating how LSD modulates "neural circuits that have been implicated in mood affective disorders, and can reduce the clinical symptoms of these disorders." According to Vollenweider and Michael Kometer, writing in *Nature*, "the controversial history" of LSD creates certain problems, although findings nonetheless raise the possibility of "promising new treatment approaches" during further investigations in "well-controlled clinical studies."[74] The work in Switzerland and the United States also harkened back to earlier questions about LSD and psychedelics – that is, about their impact on spiritual experiences and brain development. For Vollenweider, a drug-induced transcendent peak (or mystical experience) and its integration in the psychotherapeutic process might be the "crucial mechanism that enables neuroplasticity and behavioural changes."[75] In short, with technological advances in neuroimaging, as well as increased willingness on the part of regulators to sanction trials, there are encouraging opportunities ahead for scientists conducting inquiries into LSD.

Vollenweider's work in Switzerland has progressed, in part, due to more relaxed regulations concerning LSD and other hallucinogens. As Nicolas Langlitz shows, the rigours of modern lab-based research are not necessarily conducive to questions of spirituality or even consciousness as described by psychedelic encounters; indeed the psychedelic research questions of the twenty-first century are somewhat different from their 1950s counterparts. One of Langlitz's illustrative examples involves comparing psychedelic reactions between subjects who had been administered LSD and subjects who had reached a similar state of consciousness through meditation. Using brain imaging techniques and questionnaires, Vollenweider attempted to compare these experiences, but encountered a number of difficulties in securing subjects. These challenges were reminiscent of earlier psychedelic studies in the 1960s, but Vollenweider further explained how the now well-established mantra of randomized controlled trial methodology all but paralyzes such attempts to raise what are essentially philosophical and spiritual questions in brain science.

California-based neuroscientist Mark Geyer has established one of the most successful labs for investigating the effects of hallucinogens on animal behaviour. Here too the culture of modern science is brought to bear on the design of his experiments. Geyer explained to Langlitz that the historical standing of psychedelics in California has shaped the research methods, and meant that their work has centred exclusively on animal testing to satisfy regulators and ethicists. While animal models are instructive, the design also introduces certain constraints if the objective is to interrogate the way that spirituality works in the brain. Staff in Geyer's lab seemed less motivated by these bigger questions of mysticism or philosophy and instead more focused on the thorough, incremental buildup of data that can be gleaned from behavioural studies. Psychedelic drugs in that setting are merely one of many substances being tested on rodents (rats in this case). Taking time to ponder the crossroads of spirituality, consciousness, and brain science seems to have moved beyond the grasp of even the most successful researchers, whose time is increasingly devoted to securing grants, filling out ethics forms, and logging hours in the lab accumulating data. In other words, the context of modern scientific enterprises has refocused attention on data accrual and away from larger questions of ontology.

Questions concerning LSD's recent career phase now abound. In particular, there has been some skepticism about the recommencement of LSD as an object of study and the ensuing attention lavished upon it. First, a segment of the press and scientific community have challenged the "comeback" narrative. In 2006, there was certainly weight behind this statement, since there were no human studies using LSD at the time, and even if one accepts that there has been a comeback of a sort, supporters have cautiously noted that it has been a "slow revival."[76] Second, LSD has been described as a "dirty drug," recognized by critics as not only "notoriously bitchy and moody" but also imprecise compared to other psychedelics.[77] Mental health professionals who have self-experimented with LSD in this new phase, for example, have exhibited cautious attitudes about its use in therapy. In a study based in the Czech Republic, there was "lack of agreement" about whether it was possible to "eliminate the potential harm to a person during the LSD experience, even when conducting a diligent psychological examination beforehand, controlling conditions in the setting, and providing care during and after the experience."[78] Vollenweider himself has suggested that more work has to be done on both "structure-activity relationships" and the role of psychotherapeutic approaches on the effects of psychedelics to ultimately improve the benefits and minimize "unwanted side effects."[79]

As the context of psychedelic research shifts under the weight of economic austerity and, arguably, a somewhat anti-intellectual climate that forces researchers into a data-driven exercise motivated by grant-writing and impact-factor-seeking gratification, we are left to wonder whether a psychedelic renaissance is indeed underway. The comparatively more sanitized LSD research now taking place may yield important results, but we may also be forced to ask fundamentally different questions. It remains unclear whether the answers will allow us to celebrate the career of Hofmann's "problem child" or finally put the rascal to bed.

These issues were elucidated in PBS *Newshour*'s January 2017 report on the "renaissance" in psychedelics research. Studies indicating that "a single dose of psilocybin reliably helped 60 to 80 percent of [patients] feel better immediately, and for as long as six months" conveyed the promise of these once-banned compounds. But researchers did not want viewers to get the wrong idea. Dr Stephen Ross, of the NYU School of Medicine, asserted: "We're following the data. We don't think that this is going to cure anything or change the world. We are focused on helping sick people and just doing more science and following the data, seeing where it leads." Dr Michael Mithoefer was even more circumspect: "This seems to be a very powerful tool, but it's only a tool ... I think there is the danger of people thinking of it as a magic bullet."[80] Just how receptive the public is to their message of caution is muddy. The enthusiasm with which the media reports on the subject suggests there is a huge demand for mind-altering substances, despite the lack of determinative research establishing their clinical effectiveness.

CIVILIZING CANNABIS IN CANADA

In 2014–16, American and Canadian health authorities were forced to further address the issue of medical marijuana, even as activist groups and industry sought to influence the decision-making process and its place in the medical marketplace. Judging from recent developments in Canada, Mexico, and the United States, it seems we're on the edge of a transformational shift in North American drug policy. The "war on drugs" paradigm and its requisite enforcement agencies appear under greater – and more sustained – attack than perhaps ever before. This is especially true for marijuana prohibition. In Canada, medical marijuana has been widely available for more than a decade, while Prime Minister Justin Trudeau repeatedly promised to move toward a system of recreational legalization. In Mexico, the Supreme Court recently stated that individuals should have the right to grow and distribute marijuana for personal use, potentially paving the way for legal challenges to the nation's current drug laws. In the United States, likewise, more than half the states allow some degree of access to medical marijuana, with four states also providing a legal market for recreational marijuana and others primed to follow. The road forward, however, is anything but free and clear. If history acts as a guidebook, there's a great deal of haziness ahead for both the medicalization and the legalization of marijuana.[1]

In Canada, cannabis was first made illegal in 1923. By the 1960s, interest groups – including university student associations, physicians, and others – began demanding changes to the Narcotics Control Act, which governed the legal status of drugs, to decriminalize or legalize the possession of marijuana. When parliamentarians examined the provisions of the Food and Drugs Act in 1969, they asked for a special committee to look into the issue of drug use in Canada, particularly the use of cannabis. On 29 May 1969, the Liberal government headed by Pierre Elliott Trudeau passed Order-in-Council P.C. 1969-1112, establishing the Commission of Inquiry into the Non-Medical Use of Drugs. It was commonly known as the Le Dain Commission, named after its chairman, Gerald Le Dain, but was also composed of four other members: Marie-Andrée Bertrand, Ian L. Campbell, Heinz Lehman, and Peter Stein. At the time Le Dain himself was dean of Osgoode Hall in Toronto, one of the preeminent law schools in Canada, whereas Heinz Lehmann was a renowned psychiatrist at McGill University and at the forefront of treating, rather than institutionalizing, people with mental illness. Le Dain was a close friend of Prime Minister Trudeau and did not have significant experience in the field of drug law. By contrast, Dr Lehman was a world-renowned psychiatrist and scholar of substances, and had even learned through experiential research. He told a press conference that he had tried marijuana, "just as I have tried every other soft drug in the practice of my profession."[2] (Other members were quick to note that they *did not* have such experience.) Ian Campbell was arts dean at Sir George Williams University and Marie-Andrée Bertrand was a criminologist at the Université de Montréal. Peter Stein, an American who had been in Canada for six years, spent time working with prisoners across Canada in addition to treating drug users as part of the John Howard Society in Vancouver.

One of the reasons put forward to justify the Commission's creation was that the incidence of possession and use of the substances for non-medical purposes had increased, and the need for an investigation was imperative. Members noted, both individually and as a group, the lack of credible information about "soft" drugs. They insisted, too, that there was a "credibility gap" not just related to evidence but between the Canadian government and young people. Members suggested it was their "duty to establish the facts."[3]

To this end, the Commission carried out its activities from mid-October 1969 until 14 December 1973, when its final report was tabled. During this period, it heard from 639 groups and individuals: 295 organizations presented briefs and 43 appeared before the members of the Commission; 212 individuals made submissions and 89 gave oral presentations. Medical experts and basic scientists played a central role in the Commission's deliberations. Numerous renowned Canadian scientists concerned with the biochemical and pharmacological as well as the sociological and psychological elements

either testified personally or submitted reports. Representatives
from the Royal Canadian Mounted Police, the Addiction Research
Foundation of Ontario, the Narcotic Addiction Foundation of
British Columbia, l'Office de la Prevention et du Traitement de
l'Alcoolisme et des Autres Toxicomanies, various religious organizations, and other esteemed Canadian groups also weighed in.
Moreover, specialists and organizations from the United States submitted data and thoughts; and members of the Commission visited
western European countries, consulting with drug authorities there
and examining the European drug scene for themselves. In short, the
inquiry was international in scope.[4]

One non-Canadian who also took part was John Lennon. On 24
December 1969, Lennon offered his thoughts to the Commission's
deputies. "This is the opportunity for Canada to lead the world," the
Beatle testified. "I must say," the musician suggested, "this commission
that you've set up ... I don't know what's going on in the rest of the
world, you know, in reality, towards drugs, but this seems to be the
only one that is trying to find out what it's about with any kind of
sanity." He then questioned whether recreational use of the drug led to
apathy and moral degradation, as many believed. "We are one example of people who have experienced marijuana," Lennon said. "Are we
sitting in the mud? Are we sitting at home just smoking pot in a den
of iniquity?" He told them that he was forced to quit LSD because "it
did burn my head off," but that marijuana was a catalyst for peace.[5]
In total, the Commission held public hearings in 27 cities, including
Ottawa and the ten provincial capitals, travelling some 50,000 miles
around the country. During its term, the Commission published four
reports: an interim report (1970), a special report on cannabis (1972),
a report on treatment (1972), and a final report (1973).

The Commission published its cannabis findings in May 1973. The
final, 1,148-page report came out that December. The report identified
several areas of concern when it came to pot and health. Rumblings
from clinicians that chronic use was linked to mental disorders such
as schizophrenia troubled the commissioners. Most disconcerting of
all was the use of marijuana by adolescents, which "has, in all proba-
bility, a harmful effect on the maturing process." Aside from long-term
use, being acutely intoxicated did not appear to help when driving
or handling machinery. One's reflexes and judgment were impaired.
Despite rampant claims about cannabis inciting crime, there was
absolutely no evidence linking it to violence. Among the 239 criminal

cases RCMP brass chose to present to the commissioners, commissioners pointed out that only five involved crimes committed while stoned, and only two were violent. Marijuana also did not appear to be a "gateway" into opiates or stronger drugs; the report deemed scientific studies claiming as much "highly questionable." The commissioners found unequivocally that the harms of criminalizing marijuana – encouraging illicit markets, obliging pot smokers to engage in crime, diverting police from more important tasks – outweighed the harms of use. "There can be no doubt that the law on the books is at extreme variance with the facts," the report stated.[6] These findings stunned the Liberal government, including health minister John Munro and justice minister John Turner, among others, and analysts called the 1970 interim report "one of the most politically-explosive documents ever put before the government."[7]

By 1981, the debate had not abated. Policy-makers and physicians were still confused on the matter. Mel Gass, a Conservative from the Malpeque riding in Prince Edward Island, warned against liberalizing cannabis policy because of dangers to children. He claimed that the public would misinterpret the removal of punishment – essentially, incarceration – for marijuana-related crimes. This would result in "grave consequences." He argued that the Le Dain Commission was fundamentally in error about the drug:

> Much of what was said in the sixties and early seventies about the harmlessness of marijuana is obsolete and untrue. Over the past nine years medical opinion that marijuana "is a harmless substance" or "may be harmful" has been increasingly altered in favour of the opinion that "marijuana is harmfull." There have been significant changes in the position of the scientific community. Many prominent authorities on the subject who in the sixties and early seventies deemed marijuana harmless are now admitting how wrong they were.[8]

After illuminating how many in the medical field had recanted previous beliefs about the safety of cannabis, Gass informed the House of Commons about the recent consensus, or "what doctors and scientists are telling us today about the damaging effects of marijuana."[9] He recounted a frightening laundry list of harmful effects, including permanent brain atrophy, personality changes, and memory loss. It also contributed to lung cancer, disruption of female menstrual cycles to the point of causing infertility, stillbirths, fatigue, amotivational syndrome, and a "tendency toward magical thinking." "It is quite the list," Gass noted, and "is this what we want for our children?" Yet, apart from the medical discussion, law and order issues were also significant. According to Conservative Dan McKenzie, any changes to cannabis legislation would open "a real hornet's nest" of crime throughout the country. He was convinced that a lenient stance toward the drug would result in "crime, robbery, rape and what have you."[10]

JUMPING AHEAD, JUMPING BACK

Medical marijuana has been available in Canada since 2001, after the Federal Court of Appeal declared that sufferers from epilepsy, AIDS, cancer, and other ailments had a constitutional right to light up medical marijuana. Prohibition of this "medicine" was, in short, unconstitutional. And the government was forced into the construction of a regulatory architecture. The original regulation that allowed patients to access medical marijuana in Canada was enacted in 2001 and called the Marihuana Medical Access Regulations (MMAR). It allowed patients to possess dried marijuana flower/bud with a licence issued by the government, provided that the application was signed by a physician. A single strain of medicine was available for purchase from a single government supplier, Prairie Plant Systems, but optional licences were available for patients to grow their own plants or to designate a grower to supply medicine to them. Essentially, this enabled patients to obtain various strains whose characteristics could be better matched to the patient's condition, even as it was limited to patients who fell under two distinct classification schedules, which covered only the most severe and extreme conditions (while excluding some very common but still debilitating conditions and symptoms). What's more, the application process itself was complicated and lengthy, and total patients nationwide peaked at about 38,000 by the time the MMAR came to a close in March of 2014.[11]

The MMAR was repealed and replaced by the current Marihuana for Medical Purposes Regulations (MMPR), enacted on 1 April 2014. With this, medical marijuana was officially opened for business. And the new rules generated a craze as dozens of new entrants jumped into the marketplace. The program allowed patients to possess dried marijuana flower/bud with a prescription issued by a practising Canadian physician, and a government-issued licence was no longer required. Medicine was suddenly available from over thirty Health Canada–approved licensed producers (LPs). Edibles and concentrates were not legal for sale to medical marijuana patients; however, the Supreme Court ruled on 11 June 2015 that Canadians with a valid prescription could consume medical marijuana in other ways besides just the dried form. In short, the court enlarged the definition of medical marijuana, meaning that legal restrictions on extracts and derivatives were now gone, and brownies, cookies, teas, chocolate bars, and shakes, among various other products, were no longer illegal. The Canadian government was far from pleased. Federal health minister Rona Ambrose scolded the Supreme Court and told the press that she was "outraged" by the ruling. "Let's remember, there's only one authority in Canada that has the authority and the expertise to make a drug into a medicine and that's Health Canada," she said during a news conference.[12]

Then, on 23 June – about two weeks after the court decision – the first Health Canada–approved clinical trial of medical marijuana began patient recruitment in Saskatchewan. CanniMed, a Saskatoon-based company, ran the trial, which was aimed at osteoarthritis. Brent Zettl, the president and CEO of Prairie Plant Systems, which owns CanniMed, said: "In order for medical cannabis to become a true medicine, it requires carefully conducted trials to provide hard data." The following day, it was announced that Bedrocan and Tweed Marijuana, two of Canada's largest medical marijuana firms, would amalgamate in a roughly $60-million deal. Bedrocan has strengths in clinical research, while Tweed's consumer-oriented assets made the deal a good fit. It was immediately evident that medical cannabis was very big business for Canada. As the CEO of Tilray, Greg Engel, has written, "there is enormous potential for Canada to correct the harms caused by cannabis prohibition, generate meaningful tax revenue, protect children and establish this country as a global leader in this rapidly emerging industry."[13] As reported by the *National Post*, the merger was a "game changer" and would create a "dominant domestic player and reshape the fledgling industry."[14] This was no revelation, since recent articles in popular business magazines, including *Canadian Business Review*, *Fast Company*, and *Fortune*, have all underscored the potential economic and social value of adjustments to the legal status of marijuana, and have chronicled the sometimes fraught relationship between Canada's licensed producers and a nascent craft cannabis industry.

As of 24 August 2016, the MMPR was replaced with the Access to Cannabis for Medical Purposes Regulation (ACMPR). This new regulation included legislation that satisfied the latest Supreme Court decision to allow patients who possess a prescription from a doctor to grow their own medicine. Patients now had the option to grow it themselves or designate a third party to grow it for them, with a maximum of five outdoor plants or two indoor plants, the number of plants being determined by a formula based on the prescribed amount from the doctor. Patients, of course, still had to register with Health Canada in order to obtain a licence to grow their own medicine.

Amid all of this, the newly elected Liberal government, led by Prime Minister Justin Trudeau, promised legalization and then initiated a strategy to carry out the promise. A task force, which was established in June, took months to gather comments from local officials and the public before the Canadian Parliament drafted a measure. "It's a long process, and we're hard at it," noted Bill Blair, a Liberal Party MP and former Toronto police chief whom Trudeau has put in charge of the marijuana effort.[15] A task force was created, co-chaired by Anne McLellan and Dr Mark Ware.[16] Trudeau, for his part, made clear in very pragmatic terms what he hoped to do; he noted that he possessed two guiding principles in his push for legalizing pot, which were based on harm reduction principles, as opposed to maximizing benefits: to minimize underage access to marijuana and to reduce criminal activity surrounding the illegal marijuana trade.[17] For many, the collision of money, politics, and policing has made recreational marijuana a major test for Trudeau.[18]

The science and regulation of medical cannabis presented other problems. One of the many issues that created concern was marijuana policy for veterans, and the core problem rested with the amount of cannabis veterans were authorized to take. In 2014, Veterans Affairs doubled the amount to ten grams per day for eligible veterans. For Health Canada, this was twice the amount it considered safe. An internal Health Canada document showed that more than five grams had the potential to increase risks to the cardiovascular, pulmonary, and immune systems, as well as to psychomotor performance. It also had a chance of increasing the risk of drug dependence. The auditor general of Canada, Michael Ferguson, in conducting a review, could not find any evidence to support the decision to increase the threshold. Veterans affairs minister Kent Hehr expressed shock in March that his department lacked an "informed policy" on the use of medical cannabis, even as the number of claims by veterans for medical marijuana grew more than tenfold over the past two years. According to figures provided by Veterans Affairs, 112 veterans were reimbursed for medical marijuana in 2013–14. The following year, it was 628. By March 2016 that number had risen to 1,320.[19]

Mike Blais, president and founder of Canadian Veterans Advocacy, was abundantly clear about veterans' consumption of medical marijuana: "I think there should be no cap, and that every case should be judged on individual merit and that the doctor's prescription is paramount."

At the same time, the Canadian Forces have taken an alternative stand. In 2014, H.C. MacKay, who was then the deputy surgeon general of the Canadian Forces, made clear that "with respect to marijuana use for medical purposes, we have identified what appears to be a very significant policy divergence between Veterans Affairs Canada and Canadian Armed Forces." In short, even though Veterans Affairs was funding medical marijuana, the military's health service did not recognize it for medical use. With respect to PTSD, the Canadian Forces have also suggested there is insufficient evidence to authorize marijuana use and that it could even be detrimental to veterans' health.[20]

Another significant tug-of-war in the evolving Canadian medical marijuana drama pitted dispensaries against major growers, otherwise known as licensed producers. As the *New York Times* put it, "a lobbying battle is raging between the new entrepreneurs and the licensed medical marijuana producers, who were the only ones allowed to grow and provide the plant under the old regulations. One side complains about being shut out by a politically connected cartel, while the other complains about unfair and damaging competition from those who are breaking the law."[21] When the Harper Conservatives privatized the industry, they mandated delivery only by parcel post or to a doctor. Domestic "grow-ops" were outlawed. Yet, these buttoned-up regulations, according to *The Economist*, did not account for the popularity of storefront shops. Rather than passively receiving delivery by post, many consumers – both patients and partiers – obtained their marijuana through storefront "dispensaries," which sprang up across Canada, encouraged by liberalization in the United States. Traditionally, Vancouver has had the liveliest retail sector in Canada, with 176 dispensaries, or "compassion clubs," which bought the surplus produced by home-based herbalists. In the years ahead, these hope to become the basis of a legal distribution network.[22]

In Saskatoon, Saskatchewan, such hopes were put to the test in 2015, when the struggle between illegal marijuana dispensaries and licensed producers pitted the "outsiders" against the mainstream medical marijuana industry. The dispensaries – various stores, headshops, and clubs – were illegal because they procured and sold their products literally *outside* the federal medical marijuana system, which had been overhauled and expanded to allow industrial-scale production of pot products to be mailed directly to licensed patients. The entrepreneurial and combative Mark Hauk, who briefly operated Saskatoon's first medical marijuana dispensary, believed that he offered a significant face-to-face service to help "sick people in our community get access to the medicine to which they are lawfully entitled: people who have had access to their medicine blocked and are suffering needlessly, often with significant pain."[23] He opened for business on 19 August 2015, and pushback came almost immediately from national and local law enforcement, but also from the Canadian Medical Cannabis Industry Association. Prairie Plant Systems, the original sole provider in Canada, was a member of this trade association and Brent Zettl, the company's president, took issue with dispensaries, such as the one in Saskatoon. "If we were having a discussion on whether or not to open up a dispensary for fentanyl or unknown sources of OxyContin, we wouldn't be having this debate," he noted.[24] Local law enforcement officials, including the police chief in Saskatoon, Clive Weighill, who also happened to be the head of the Canadian Association of Municipal Police Chiefs, stated that he was "working with Health Canada and the federal prosecutions on this."[25] The bullish Hauk argued that threats wouldn't close his pot club. After his club received a notice from Health Canada warning of possible RCMP raids, the fate of his dispensary was sealed. It was raided on 29 October and shut down, actions he called "nothing short of shameful and gutless."[26] (What Hauk may or may not have known was that Saskatoon had one of the highest enforcement rates for cannabis possession in Canada and a long history of anti-marijuana sentiments tied to the US War on Drugs.[*27])

---

* Eloise Opheim was executive director of PRIDE-CANADA, a national organization based in Saskatoon aimed at limiting drug use.

What is most fascinating about this from a historical perspective is how many of these issues have a familiar ring. Physicians and pharmacists wrote of the potential dangers of cannabis almost immediately following its formal introduction to American medicine in the 1840s. Most medical doctors understood that cannabis was both potentially helpful and potentially harmful. These concerns stemmed from the adverse events and feelings that sometimes accompanied the use of cannabis medicines, including distortions of space and time, hallucinations, anxiety, and fear of death. While some of the physicians' anxiety was attributed to high variability in the potency of cannabis from plant to plant and product to product, the mode of administration also surely helped. There are a few scattered references to cannabis smoking among nineteenth-century Americans, but most cannabis preparations were consumed in more concentrated liquid or edible form.

Hauk, too, resembled Judith Quattlebaum, Ron Woodroof, or Jenny McCarthy, in that he was confronting the power structure of drug regulation, including licensed producers in the province. As cannabis was increasingly pharmaceuticalized and the industry consolidated to a greater extent, Hauk offered a service that resided outside of the governing structure. He represented the activism and entrepreneurialism, the fringe, perhaps even quackery. His business operated on the periphery of the mainline medical cannabis industry, and ultimately challenged the newly emerging marijuana companies. (In doing so, he strongly denied that he was catering to recreational users or "stoners.") Hauk was essentially playing the role of McConaughey in his own Saskatoon Buyers Club. And this sequel acts as a reminder about the complexity of modern drug regulation in modern Canadian society, as well as the ways in which everyday citizens can both run afoul of the regulatory system *and* potentially influence it.

RESEARCH DILEMMAS AND DEFICIENCIES

Canadian physicians were given the primary authority in authorizing legal access to cannabis in 2016. One physician described the role as that of a gatekeeper.[28] However, this role did not sit well with many doctors for multiple reasons. To begin with, because of "a lack of robust supporting published evidence, personal reasons, and advice from multiple associations, many physicians were reluctant to authorize this remedy."[29] Similarly, as other chapters of this book have shown, doctors were placed in a difficult position by the demands for a strange medicine and the medico-scientific evidence about the safe and effective use of the treatment. In the case of cannabis, these demands emanated from the courts, the public, and beyond; it should come as no great surprise, either, that medical authorities in Canada resisted the government's delegation of responsibility and the legal system's passing of the proverbial buck. This back and forth – the tension over the regulation of a given drug – was evident with medical heroin, for instance.

Then, as now, various medical constituencies commented on the legitimacy of cannabis and, more particularly, cannabinoids. The Canadian Medical Association opposed Health Canada's approach to widening access to medical cannabis. For example, the CMA specified that physicians should not feel pressured to authorize marijuana for medical purposes; meanwhile, any physician who chose to authorize marijuana had to comply with provincial or territorial regulatory College's relevant guideline or policy. One wonders why they would not. The CMA further questioned "the serious lack of clinical research, guidance and regulatory oversight for marijuana as a treatment."[30] To shape the terms of debate, the CMA offered recommendations about cannabis. Two of these included limiting payments from patients for this service and the need for follow-up consultations.

Other groups and organizations got involved in the discussion as well. The College of Family Physicians of Canada argued that Health Canada's regulations put family physicians in a challenging spot, one where they were asked to authorize their patient's access to a product with little evidence to support its use, and in lieu of regulatory oversight and approval. The CFPC suggested this was "unfair," "untenable," and "unethical."[31] Provincial bodies that govern medical practice and physicians, called Colleges of Physicians and Surgeons, also created medical cannabis bylaws and guidelines. Evidence and research often served as bases for these rules. British Columbia's College of Physicians and Surgeons held that "few reliable published studies are available on the benefits of marijuana in smoked form." It continued: "many uncertainties remain about the effects, both beneficial and harmful, of smoked marijuana."[32] In Saskatchewan, the College of Physicians and Surgeons underlined that the limited scientific and clinical assessment made safe authorization nigh on impossible, despite what the federal government regulations allowed for.

Much like LSD in its earliest years, then, marijuana has riveted the minds of clinical, bio-medical, spiritual, and political thinkers criss-crossing the disciplines. For some, the majority of the research on cannabinoid agents has been associated with particular pharmaceutical medications, such as nabilone capsules (Cesamet) and nabiximols oral spray (Sativex). For others, the hype surrounding medical cannabis has grown so intense that it has prompted a satirical counterattack, as in Vann R. Newkirk II's article "What Can't Medical Marijuana Do?"[33] The drug's unconventional – outsider – status has meant that it has become an object of both derision and admiration. Physicians, accordingly, have been split. Many have opted to authorize the use of cannabis; others, meanwhile, have chosen not to use a substance without clear evidence about the risks, benefits, potential complications, and drug interactions.

Cannabis policy in the United States, according to one prominent pharmacologist, has largely been directed by lawmakers and law enforcement. Scientists "have had virtually no say" in the matter and their work has been "completely overlooked" when it "didn't happen to fit in with [the government's] political position."[34] Similarly, scientists and physicians have played second fiddle in Canada, and have been directed by politicians, policy-makers, the judiciary, and citizens leading the cannabis debate. After thousands were arrested during the 1960s, when the government cracked down on cannabis users, Canadians pressured government to do something about the "many young, middle-class offenders" whose records were marred by cannabis-related criminal convictions. This led to the Le Dain Commission's recommendation of decriminalization in the early 1970s, after which nothing of consequence was immediately done.[35] Support for the legalization of cannabis exploded once more when Liberal leader Justin Trudeau made it a signature part of his 2015 election campaign and the promise served as one of several reasons he won in a landslide. Drug laws have criminalized an estimated 500,000 to 1.5 million Canadians and, indeed, Canada has had one of the highest rates of cannabis usage in the world.[36] Proposals for liberalization of cannabis laws in Canada have also resulted not simply from the findings of the medical establishment, but from the agitation of activists, governmental prohibition fatigue, and the fact of cannabis's recreational popularity. Trudeau, a former snowboard instructor and onetime *bon vivant*, himself admitted to smoking cannabis while he was a sitting MP.[37] Of his history with cannabis,

he said: "Sometimes, I guess, I have gotten a buzz, but other times
no. I'm not really crazy about it."[38]

Most importantly, the loosening of restrictions on "medical marijuana" in 2001 served as "the 'sneaky side-door' towards cannabis control reform."[39] In short, Canadian citizens were accustomed
to the legal consumption of cannabis – at least in a medical sense
– when the Liberals propounded the prospect of full-scale legalization. In 2016, the Canadian government reiterated many of the
points made in the Le Dain Commission's 1973 report. Prohibition,
it determined once more, fuelled crime, generated high costs for the
police, judiciary, and corrections service, and inhibited access to
medical treatment. It also failed categorically: in 2013, 11 percent of
Canadians, or 3.1 million individuals, admitted to consuming marijuana.[40] Not surprisingly, this has frustrated drug-takers who see
little harm in cannabis use. Those caught possessing the drug illicitly
have characterized the enforcement of the legal regime as arbitrary
and depending "on the attitude of the cop who catches" you.[41] Many
youth do not understand why it is even policed, especially since cannabis is prescribed by doctors, and drug paraphernalia, from bongs
to vaporizers, are widely and legally available.[42] Indeed, many young
people do not consider cannabis to be a drug on par with alcohol
or tobacco.[43] Such hypocrisy and inconsistency has also changed the
way the public views cannabis. If Justin Trudeau can smoke cannabis and get away with it, why can't regular Canadians? And though
government and the public have come around to the idea of legalizing, taxing, and regulating cannabis in the same way as alcohol and
tobacco,[44] many public health officials and some politicians are concerned that the push to legalize it is motivated by market-imperative
and libertarian considerations rather than the scientific evidence.[45]
Such critics may be right.

Testifying before a government committee, Hillary Geller, assis-
tant deputy minister at Health Canada, submitted that cannabis was
legalized "for medical purposes in response to a decision made by the
courts." It was a legal determination, rather than a scientific one, that
gave patients access to cannabis in the first place. Health Canada,
she argued, had not approved cannabis as a "drug or medicine" and
"dried marijuana has not gone through the clinical trials, etc., and the
rigorous process that is required for any other prescription medication in this country."[46] Physicians supported this stance in the main,
not wanting to risk their patients' health before sufficient studies had

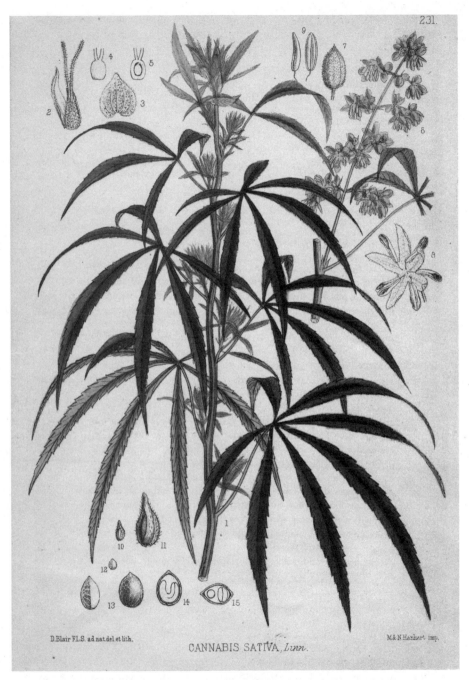

FIGURE 5.1 Cannabis sativa. In *Medicinal Plants*, v. IV, no. 231. Rockville, MD. Collections of the National Library of Medicine.

been carried out.[47] For instance, family physicians were advised as late as 2014 to avoid prescribing smoked cannabis except in instances where patients had not "responded to standard analgesics and synthetic cannabinoids" in the treatment of their "severe neuropathic pain." In brief, the insufficient evidence establishing cannabis's efficacy, and no definitive guideline on prescribing it, has led authorities to counsel caution.[48] As such, Health Canada refrained from supporting medical claims in its 2013 packet of *Information for Health Care Professionals*: "This document should not be construed as expressing conclusions from Health Canada about the appropriate use of cannabis (marihuana) or cannabinoids for medical purposes."[49] Consumers have been warned, too, that "[c]annabis is not an approved therapeutic product" and "[t]he use of this product involves risks to health, some of which may not be fully understood."[50]

Messages, that is, about the risks and rewards of cannabis haven't been effectively communicated on a number of fronts. Some perceive cannabis as a "natural product" that might "prevent or cure cancer."[51] Rectifying these misconceptions and warning individuals of the risks of cannabis use has proven difficult. Experts have stated that there is a link between cannabis use and schizophrenia "among some vulnerable groups" "though [it is] not well understood."[52] As Matthew Hill noted: "It is important to ensure we do not confuse correlation with causation [in the cannabis and schizophrenia research debate] and incite another *Reefer Madness*."[53] Links of this kind need to be sorted out. Scare tactics will only make things worse.

Nowhere in this narrative does the scientific evidence feature prominently. On the contrary, the absence of scientific evidence is glaring. As one critic of legalization put it: "any decision to legalize cannabis in Canada now cannot really be 'evidence-based' and must rest primarily on broader social values, ideals and hopes" or be "driven by ideology."[54] The evolution in values – and the role of the judiciary – is what has led to the proposed legalization of cannabis, not the facts. A survey of twenty-eight studies on the social effects of the use of cannabis for therapeutic purposes determined that more data are needed "to direct and assess policy changes with scientific data, instead of plain beliefs or misconceptions."[55] Not only is the medical science inadequate to mandate legalization, the social science is indeterminate as well.

The available proof has done little to alter deeply entrenched attitudes towards cannabis. The Canadian Medical Association (CMA) has been criticized for its opposition to medical cannabis. One group of researchers has claimed that the CMA has failed "to acknowledge various peer-reviewed and high-quality clinical research studies on the therapeutic application of cannabis," making their view "not entirely evidence-based."[56] Just how much it will take for an organization such as the CMA to change its tune remains an open question, but its position is not anti-science nor wholly ideological. There is insufficient evidence to back many of the claims made by cannabis advocates. Yet, the paucity of proof establishing cannabis as an effective medical treatment has resulted in part from cannabis's status as a "highly controlled substance," making it difficult to explore its "medical and therapeutic potential."[57] Perhaps, if/when cannabis is legalized in Canada, researchers will be able to state with greater certainty the utility and harmfulness of this widely used substance. Until that time, its medical use will remain controversial. There may be growing support internationally for the study of cannabis and cannabinoids and a consensus is slowly building on their efficacy. Many investigators know they have "therapeutic potential over a wide range of non-psychiatric and psychiatric disorders such as anxiety, depression, and psychosis," but what is unknown are "the mechanisms responsible for [their] therapeutic potential."[58] Researchers admit there is a lot to be learned:

> Strong evidence supports the use of cannabinoids for chronic pain, but more research is needed to determine which diagnoses, pain characteristics, and clinical variables are most amenable to treatment; the long term effectiveness of these drugs; optimal drug selection and dosages; the risk-benefit ratio of combining cannabinoids with other drugs; and how adverse effects can be minimised.[59]

Answers to important cannabis questions will require "a political climate conducive" to this research.[60] Likewise, the medico-scientific as well as socio-political firmament has begun to shift to the idea of supporting these inquiries. The legalization and/or decriminalization of cannabis in the Netherlands, several US states, and Uruguay, along with liberal or liberalizing regimes in Canada, Spain, and Germany, has illustrated that cannabis is increasingly considered a part of modern medicine. What public health officials and doctors do not know, though, creates suspicion. Perhaps the debate has moved too rapidly? What of cannabis's effect on developing brains? How will "drug-driving" be policed? Myriad other questions need answering. Finally, as one worried commentator put it: "How do we keep it away from kids? The pot pushers – the politicians and marijuana marketers – now need to step up and help do it, as they promised."[61]

THEY MEAN BUSINESS

The federal government has regulated access to medical cannabis since 2001, but between that year and 2015 a paltry two clinical studies received federal funding to investigate its medicinal value. Austerity and governments averse to raising cannabis's profile – particularly the Conservative governments of Stephen Harper – partially led to the lack of data. The result is that scientists have to play catch-up to policy-makers. As Jonathan Page and Mark Ware put it: "The science of medical cannabis desperately needs to get out in front of policy. It would be unforgivable if ten years from now we are still lamenting the lack of research despite widespread access to medical cannabis and a profit-hungry industry."[62] A real risk exists that "Big Cannabis" and the market imperative will overtake public health considerations and, though cannabis will be regulated, it could cause harm as well as succour – as has happened with the commercialization of alcohol, tobacco, and sugar.[63] Some evidence suggests that this will happen. A windfall in tax revenue for governments has been part of the draw for liberalizers and will certainly prove alluring in the future. Public health commentators urge that this revenue should be spent on prevention through education, research, and access to treatment.[64] Accordingly, "What Can't Marijuana Do?" is not the only pressing question. Just as important is "What Can't Marijuana Fund?" Countless individuals, organizations, and companies will profit from cannabis, including the government, and part of the dividend will be allocated to combatting the negative consequences of legalization. Or so the public has been told. The interests of the nascent "Big Cannabis" are antithetical to the civilizing of cannabis.

Many physicians remain skeptical of anecdotal evidence about cannabis as "a viable therapeutic option," especially since much of this data derives from private producers "investing in research to add credibility to their products." The CEO of BioMed, Justin Dhaliwal, believes cannabis will "improve the lives of Canadians" and that the industry has a "duty to go ahead and spend the money in research to show that evidence."[65] A familiar story in drug history, such language about safety and efficacy has cut across the spectrum of preventive and palliative medicine, from Laetrile to heroin and beyond. Tobacco-funded research sought to prove their product was not as harmful as public health officials contended; and it took decades for the push-back to reduce the number of users, thereby mitigating the harm tobacco caused. "Big Cannabis," when placed in the history of substances and medicines, will likely play a familiar role. It certainly will not be any less induced to maximize its profits, no matter the social cost. ArcView Market Research calculated that Canadians and Americans spent a total of $72 billion Canadian (US $56.4 billion) on cannabis in 2016. This estimate was based on medicinal, legal, and illegal sale figures.[66] That is a big market, with plenty of room for expansion. It remains an intriguing question whether legislators can resist the temptations of a likely revenue windfall and prioritize public health. Early indications from the United States suggest private interests will win the day. The regulatory models in place in Colorado and Washington put profits before public health.*[67] The harms of cannabis, relative to such other products as alcohol or powerful painkillers, will need to be addressed in this deliberation as well.

Business leaders are pushing for a market-oriented approach in Canada, too. The Saskatchewan-born oil and gas entrepreneur Brett Wilson has invested millions in the cannabis industry, which has grown "at a frenetic pace." He claims he "wants to accelerate research into marijuana's medicinal properties while promoting what he calls responsible consumption." To this end, he invested in Vancouver's Tokyo Smoke, a company with aspirations to "become the Starbucks of cannabis."[68] Whether a Starbucks-style corporation will invest in research that could potentially undermine its product's safety and reputation remains to be seen. But Wilson and others are betting that cannabis will go mainstream. The battle for celebrity endorsements has already begun, with rapper Snoop Dogg signing on to work with Tweed Inc. of Smith Falls, Ontario in 2016. Snoop was excited to work with the pot producer, saying: "Canada has been at the forefront of the business model, and I look forward to being a part of the road

---

* For example, limits on advertising are based on those placed on the alcohol industry, many of which are voluntary or vague.

ahead." He also noted how attitudes have changed: "There are real
social and medical benefits from the cannabis industry, and the world
is seeing this positivity in a whole new way."[69]

The Centre for Addiction and Mental Health (CAMH) has also contributed to the discussion about the business of cannabis. According
to CAMH, cannabis has been "viewed through a law enforcement lens"
and a transition towards a "public health approach" will be crucial
in the years ahead.[70] Preventing harm should be the focus of the latter.[71] Using alcohol and tobacco as examples, CAMH warned against
letting the market "push the boundaries of health-focused regulation."
Over time and space advocates for these two substances, because of
immense profitability, have been able to fight governmental attempts
at regulation, despite indisputable social harm. When "Big Cannabis"
has "an incentive to find new customers, retain existing ones, and
encourage high levels of consumption," the authorities should be
concerned. To elude the historical excesses found in the alcohol and
tobacco industries, Canada will need to "pre-empt [the] conflict that
exists between public health goals and the profit motive."[72] CAMH
expressed hope that the government would resist the temptations of
embarrassing riches and establish a sensible cannabis policy that bal-
ances the interests of public health with those of individual rights and
the free market. At the same time, responding to criticisms of their
research paper on the ideological production and use of evidence in
the cannabis policy debate, Macleod and Hickman recently indicated
data were abundant enough to justify the promulgation of policies
aimed at limiting cannabis consumption.[73] More scientific information was needed, they suggested, yet "we seem to have come to a
point where we can agree on the list" of health risks.[74] More data
was required about cannabis and cannabinoids as an effective therapy. Until this has been done, those who believe cannabis works will
continue to tout its benefits, opponents characterizing it as a social
harm will decry its proliferation, and experts will lament their lack of
knowledge. Industry will cash in amid this process.

During the twentieth century, Big Tobacco engaged in a commercial, cultural, and scientific battle to convince the medical establishment and public that its product was first healthful and thereafter
innocuous.[75] This message became increasingly difficult to sustain
as citizens grew ill in greater numbers and perceptions of tobacco
transformed. Hence, the industry modified its position. Throughout
the 1950s, and into the 1970s, Big Tobacco employed scientific

research to displace its product as the primary cause of diseases associated with and attributed to tobacco use. It pointed the finger at genetics in the etiology of tobacco-related ailments rather than tobacco or nicotine per se.[76] These hazy obfuscations were illuminated once the data established as fact that tobacco caused cancer and many other illnesses. What some critics of cannabis legalization fear is that a similar process will be enacted, and that we just don't know enough about this strange medicine to be sure that it is harmless.[*][77] Statements suggesting thousands of deaths may be caused by increased access to cannabis, for example, have been criticized for drawing a tendentious parallel between cannabis and tobacco.[78] The largest study on the effects of cannabis and cannabinoids to date suggests "that smoking cannabis does not increase the risk of certain cancers."[79] Even so, what about the effects that are not yet known? Determinations about the safety and efficacy of cannabis are far from a conclusion. Of course, those in the cannabis industry want us to believe it isn't harmful and ought to be considered a therapy or medicine; they will profit from its sale. In the case of cannabis, then, a balance will need to be struck between prudent caution and regurgitation of an updated version of *Reefer Madness*.

---

* "The challenge facing policymakers and public health advocates is reducing the harms of ... [the] 'war on drugs' while preventing another public health catastrophe similar to tobacco use, which kills 6 million people worldwide each year."

Part Three

DEMONIZED PHARMACEUTICALS

THE "MAPLE PERIL" AND THE WAR ON TERROR: PHARMACEUTICAL PURCHASING IN THE WAKE OF SEPTEMBER 11

American pharmaceutical products under patent are, for the most part, much more expensive than Canadian ones, which has prompted savvy American consumers to purchase theirs abroad. These bargain-hunters have shopped online, through internet pharmacies, and also the old-fashioned way, taking bus trips across the border to fill prescriptions in Canadian pharmacies. As this practice grew in scope from the mid-1990s, the issue also grew more politically charged. The idea that drugs from Canada – even though approved and occasionally manufactured in the US – were circumventing profits and safety nets gained momentum. Various parties raised red flags. This type of medical tourism was not the same as Steve McQueen's visits to Mexico, because travellers were not seeking out underground, alternative medicines. No, the drugs purchased by Americans in Canada were FDA-approved and manufactured by multinational companies. The products were not strange medicines. Laetrile was illegal. Statins and beta-blockers were legal, and mainstream. The following pages chart how key actors, including Congress, the bureaucrats in the US and Canada, activist groups, and the pharmaceutical industry, changed the perceptions of many legitimate drugs. How were approved pharmaceuticals portrayed? And why? This chapter is a mere snapshot and doesn't focus on single products. There are excellent studies on how approved pharmaceuticals, such as thalidomide, Oraflex, Prozac, or Vioxx, were recalled from the market and saw their 'careers' take dramatic turns. The intention here, however, is to stimulate a wider discussion about pharmaceutical products.[1]

At the end of the 1990s and at the outset of the new millennium, US drug industry officials argued that the practice of "reimportation"

– Americans taking a trip to Canada or ordering drugs online – was hazardous to Americans and destabilized companies' ability to finance crucial research and development. Major drug firms contended that in the long run this posed a threat to American patients and consumers. Two overriding concerns dominated: the loss of revenue and loss of accountability. These drugs, once shipped abroad, fell outside the zone of American regulation and constituted a danger to Americans' health. Terrorists and other sorts of criminals, it was alleged, might use this security loophole to attack the US, which prompted Harvard scholar Jerry Avorn to call the demonization of pharmaceuticals from Canada a "maple peril."[2] Approved drugs were demonized. The cross-border pharmaceutical trade between two friendly neighbours created a rift. This matters because it reveals how pharmaceutical products – approved and manufactured in the US – could gravitate from the realm of acceptability to a position where they were considered risky objects. Essentially, they migrated from a position of acceptance to a position of strangeness, where they were characterized similarly to recreational drugs such as heroin, Laetrile, or LSD; President George W. Bush, for example, made this clear during a presidential debate, when he stated, "When a drug comes in from Canada, I want to make sure it cures you and doesn't kill you."[3] An analysis of this shift – good drugs going bad – adds extra layers to the understanding of business interests, government, and health consumers in adjudicating contested medicines in the marketplace.[4] It adds to our analysis of cash and consumer safety, the use of proper evidence, and politics and personal autonomy in the medical sphere.

Ultimately, cross-border pharmaceutical drug purchasing was a thorny problem that centred on drug safety, access, and most of all, Americans' pocketbooks. Senator Debbie Stabenow (D-MI), who supported the legalization of reimportation, chastised the pharmaceutical industry for its expensive prices and the essentially unbearable costs that forced Americans to buy their drugs abroad. (In recent years, of course, Martin Shkreli, EpiPens, and President Donald Trump have reignited the discussion.[5]) She asserted, then, that Big Pharma had a "stranglehold on the U.S. consumer."[6] In the mid-1990s the Clinton administration first grappled with the flow of prescription drugs from Canada, eventually resisting attempts to legalize the practice. When President Bush took office, he also wrestled with the complex financial and safety imperatives of the so-called "maple peril," to say nothing of the creeping fear of socialized medicine. As had occurred under the

Clinton administration, members of Bush's own party, politicians such as Senator John McCain (R-AZ), challenged the status quo and pushed for solutions to the issue. At various times, Bush even seemed amenable to legalization and highlighted his openness to Canadian drugs approved for use in the United States. Despite his rhetoric, though, the political reality was that he sought to stem the flow of Canadian drugs into the United States, not increase it.[7]

By 1994, there was a larger shift in American politics itself. A "conservative paradigm" continued to direct the period and the "Republican revolution" of 1994 was a vital part of the relationship between the pharmaceutical industry and the FDA. More specifically, during the 1994 midterm elections, a ferociously antigovernment variety of Republicans led by Representative Newt Gingrich of Georgia won majorities in both the House and Senate. His "Contract with America" demonized President Clinton, promised to end the "scandal and disgrace" of the Democratic Congress, and clearly delineated small government and antiregulatory principles. According to David Halberstam, the conservative right wing which had spawned this contract were the "children of the Reagan revolution now coming of age, driven by their own passions and, like many true believers before them, accustomed to talking only with people who agreed with them."[8] "They were deeply distrustful," equally, "of the very government that they, like it or not, were now an important part of."[9] The FDA, amid this revolution, had once again become a "lightning rod for antigovernment sentiments," forcing Commissioner Kessler to comment, "It's not fashionable to be a regulator these days."[10]

The FDA's pharmaceutical policies, which constituted part of what the new breed of conservatives deemed an intrusive and overbearing government, were especially singled out for demonization. Speaker Gingrich called the FDA the nation's "number one job-killer" and underlined a desperate need for FDA reform.[11] By 1995, a full-scale anti-FDA campaign was underway, with conservative pundit James Brosvard encapsulating the struggle: "One of the clearest tests of whether a Republican Congress can begin to rein in big government will be the ... battle over the future of the FDA."[12] Yet, both patient-consumer groups and the pharmaceutical industry demonstrated a degree of division and reluctance about a wholesale change of drug policies at the agency. For example, the Patient Coalition, a collection of patient groups, articulated strident support of the FDA, whereas the Public Citizen's Dr Sidney Wolfe, who had made a career out of criticizing the agency, warned of the dangers weakening the agency. In contrast, "phony grassroots groups" represented another patient-consumer opinion, as patients and families were flown into Washington specifically for the FDA reform debate. Their message, according to Philip J. Hilts, aligned with the "hard right" Republican view: Americans were dying of red tape – much like Laetrile advocates had suggested in the early 1980s – and the FDA ought to be dismantled.[13]

The pharmaceutical industry, for its part, struck an uneasy balance between support for the FDA and attempts at reform. The Pharmaceutical Research and Manufacturers Association (PhRMA), which represented all drug-makers in the United States, was placed in a peculiar position where it advocated "quantum changes" in FDA operations, but also sought to prevent significant and irreparable damage to the agency.[14] "Drug companies were doing well – business was good and getting better, profits were high, the FDA was moving faster than ever – but the companies had no desire to alienate the new Republican leadership."[15] It consequently allied with such groups as the Cato Institute, Citizens for a Sound Economy, the Progress and Freedom Foundation, and the Washington Legal Foundation, which had competed with each other in 1995–96 to produce and promote radical FDA reform measures. At the same time, the pharmaceutical industry did not entirely accept "conservative mythology" and often publicly employed softer terms such as transformation and bipartisanship when discussing possible changes at the FDA.[16] PhRMA president Alan Holmer publicly announced that the industry wanted "consensus" and "noncontroversial FDA modernization."[17]

Efforts for FDA reform reached their zenith in 1996. Representative Ron Wyden (D-OR) introduced an omnibus bill in 1995 that would have expedited the drug approval process and strengthened the role of outside advisory panels, though it failed to gain traction. The following year, Senator Nancy Kassebaum (R-KA) proposed a bill to achieve the same outcome: she incorporated a six-month deadline for FDA action on NDAS (new drugs applications), a 120-day deadline for approval of drugs to treat life-threatening illnesses or those for which no other treatment existed, and a provision that allowed UK- or EU-approved products on the American market. In the House of Representatives, Thomas Bliley (R-VA) possessed an alternative vision of FDA reform. Earlier in the year, the Progress &

Freedom Foundation (PFF), which had strong ties to Gingrich's office, unveiled a new plan for FDA reform that included privatizing and eliminating the agency's gatekeeping powers through "third party" reviewers.[18] These outside reviewers, designated as Drug and Device Certification Bodies (DCBs), would essentially serve as independent bodies advising manufacturers on the design and conduct of trials and FDA rules.* Representative Bliley, for his part, was very much in support of this type of solution to what he perceived as the FDA's problems. Consequently, the legislative efforts in 1996 sought to streamline the FDA drug approval process, through either rigid time limits on FDA action or outsourcing some of the decision-making.

During committee hearings in 1996, the anti-FDA sentiments were front and centre and the debate over consumer choice and sound FDA regulation created considerable publicity. Commissioner Kessler, for his part, regarded the Bliley bill and the hearings themselves as potentially dangerous for Americans. "This is as serious as it gets," he told one reporter the day of his testimony.[19] From the opening statement, the FDA found itself on the defensive. Vilified for its slow approval times and denying sick Americans life-saving drugs, the FDA was portrayed in the broadest strokes possible, but also as solely culpable for delays. The nuances inherent to such an incredibly difficult task as drug approval and protection – be they the "experience" of a company in preparing an acceptable application or how the FDA fared relative to other regulatory bodies – were noticeably absent. In the face of such criticism, Kessler was unrepentant as he explained that the FDA rested at the interface of business and industry, physicians and academic researchers, patient-consumer groups, and politicians. Over several hours of testimony he carefully defended the agency, stressed its role in protecting the public health, and highlighted the unmistakable radicalism of the "reform" bills.[20]

"A MEDICATION NATION" AND "REIMPORTATION"

In recent years, we have been furnished with a vital glimpse into the role of pharmaceuticals in American society, politics, and the economic system. We have received, in short, *The Truth about*

---

* Under this law, FDA personnel would be empowered to certify the DCBs and maintain post-marketing surveillance.

Drug Companies. For instance, we have learned about the growth in disease diagnoses and definitions in the United States since the 1950s. We have learned that drug companies used the politics of the Cold War to defend themselves against damning charges made by congressional investigations, and this has enhanced our understanding of the pharmaceutical industry's part in the development of the modern American state.[21] Other writers have charted the pharmaceutical industry's relationship with drugs and narcotics, such as Miltown, LSD, marijuana, and heroin, both on the home front and abroad.[22] For historians, what's fascinating with the story of reimportation (and let's face facts, it doesn't sound overly riveting) is that even the quickest glance at the "maple peril" illustrates how pharmaceutical products – not just recreational drugs – can be bound up in fiery rhetoric, in borderline moral panics, and become demonized products themselves. In an age when prescription painkillers are dominating headlines because of tragic overdoses, this tale takes on even more salience.

Prescription and generic drugs have come to play an enormous role in Americans' lives as well as the US healthcare system, and many excellent writers, including Marcia Angell and Jeremy Greene, as well as Stan Finkelstein and Peter Temin, have chronicled this trend. *Fortune* magazine dubbed the United States a "medication nation" in 2014. In 1980, US prescription drug expenditures were $12 billion, accounting for 4.9 percent of total healthcare spending. By 2003, it had escalated to $184.1 billion or 11 percent of total healthcare spending. During the same period, prescription drug spending also increased at an annual rate of between 10 and 14 percent.[23]

Lower drug prices in Canada forged a strong relationship between American consumers and the Canadian industry, leading to the expansion of illegal cross-border reimportation. This occurred in person or through an internet pharmacy. In Canada, the Patented Medicines Price Review Board (PMPRB) enforces federal price regulations, but a number of other reasons also drive down Canadian drug prices. Lower prices on Canadian brand-name drugs are likely the normal result of market economics; that is, prices are matched to different supply and demand dynamics in the Canadian and American markets. Moreover, the bulk-purchasing power of provincial governments drives down prices in Canada, undermining the argument that price controls are the primary determinant in the cost of brand-name drugs in Canada.[24]

In 2001, Americans were saving a mind-boggling 50 percent to 70 percent filling their prescriptions in Canada, thanks to price-control regulations – as well as a weak Canadian dollar.[25] In 2004, one report suggested that Americans paid an average of 67 percent more than Canadians for patented drugs. For instance, in 2003 a three-month prescription for Merck's cholesterol reducer Zocor cost $172 in Canada and $328 in the US. The antiretroviral drug ritonavir (Norvir) cost as little as $700 per year in Canada; the price was $7,800 per year in the US.[26] For consumers it was a rational economic decision to buy cheaper Canadian drugs. And this became a vital political and economic issue for the Bush administration, which touted free markets and consumer choice. Three factors helped drive the political debate and the administration's response. First, in the 2000 elections, exorbitantly high drug costs had featured in senatorial, congressional, and gubernatorial races from Maine to California.[27] Second, by 2003 nearly two million Americans purchased their products from Canada, a practice surely fuelled by the considerable size of the uninsured population, which paid for medications out-of-pocket. Third, reimportation had a detrimental effect on US pharmaceutical sales, an industry that offered significant contributions to the Republican Party.[28]

US politicians tackled the troubling matter of drug costs in the 1950s. Historian David Herzberg, author of *Happy Pills*, argues that "increasing competition and ever more intense advertising *transformed* the character of the once-staid prescription drug business."[29] The newly changed pharmaceutical industry was challenged in the political arena when in December 1959 feisty and ambitious Senator Estes Kefauver (D-TN) took up the general issue of prices. Through the Senate Subcommittee on Antitrust and Monopoly he investigated a host of industries, including "bread, milk, auto, steel, and electrical manufacturing" industries. He also focused on the American pharmaceutical industry's monopoly – its stranglehold on the American consumer – and revealed a "series of price-fixing and collusion scandals."[30] During the ten-month hearings, a hundred and fifty witnesses testified about cortical steroids, tranquilizers, antibiotics, and oral antidiabetics. Kefauver, who "favored an economy in which competition among small producers set prices," asserted loudly and often that the drug industry practised "price leadership" and suffered little foreign or domestic competition. His two principal experts, Dr John Blair and lawyer Paul Rand Dixon, were media savvy – in an era before the 20-second sound-bite and 24-hour news cycle – and compared a drug's production costs to its wholesale and retail prices. Thereafter they brusquely questioned representatives of the pharmaceutical industry and neatly underlined the fact that consumers in the United States were paying a hefty sum for their medications. In one extraordinary example, the markup was a Martin Shkreli–like 7,000 percent.[31]

Kefauver's subcommittee hearings and the thalidomide scare in 1962 ultimately contributed to the passage of the 1962 Kefauver-Harris Act, although licensing, greater patent regulation, and pricing reforms were excluded from the final legislation. Still, Kefauver's legislation had a lasting impact: the new law established standardized manufacturing procedures and made safety and effectiveness requirements for approval. The new law was crucial; it represented a "watershed moment in the nation's approach to medications" and "completely changed the way doctors and patients thought about drugs."[32]

By the late twentieth century, a robust regulatory framework and a closed distribution system protected American drugs. Maintaining the security of the American drug supply is enormously complicated, and products from the outside – from Canada, no less – opened gaps in the ostensibly closed system. Storage and packaging conditions, the manufacturing point, and the dosage form and potency: these factors, according to the FDA, are nearly impossible to verify outside of a well-controlled, closely regulated system. This fact has led to a remarkably consistent approach from the agency's politically appointed leadership.[33] The FDA's resistance to pharmaceutical reimportation dates to 1969 and ten of the previous eleven FDA commissioners opposed reimportation legislation.[34] Yet, resistance has not been absolute. Despite the FDA's consistency in protecting the integrity of US companies, the agency adopted a benignly neglectful approach to Canadian drugs in the recent past – because they were *Canadian drugs*. The FDA exercised "enforcement discretion" on medication imports from its neighbour to the north, which essentially allowed most filled prescription drugs from Canada into the United States, provided they were intended for personal use and the supply did not exceed ninety days' worth.[35]

Money was definitely a reason underlying such "benign neglect." Sustaining the integrity of the closed distribution system requires vigilance and vast resources, and in the early years of the Bush administration it was made clear by the FDA and Customs Service and Border Patrol (CBP) that they did not have enough money or personnel to undertake comprehensive examinations of all parcels. In short, due to budget shortfalls they could not guarantee safety and security. In 2003, customs workers inspected less than 1 percent of an estimated two million packages of medicine that entered the United States. At John F. Kennedy Airport Mail Facility, which in 2003 received 40,000 packages per day suspected to contain drugs, only 500 to 700 were actually inspected. One pilot program in 2003 found that of the 1,153 packages inspected in select mail facilities in Miami, New York City, San Francisco, and Carson, CA, 88 percent contained dangerous, unapproved, or counterfeit drugs from numerous countries. Some of the unsafe drugs that originated in Canada included: (1) drugs different from those approved by the FDA; (2) drugs requiring careful dosing; (3) drugs with potential for dangerous interactions; and (4) drugs requiring screening or monitoring.[36] By the end of the Bush administration, the situation remained dire.[37]

Counterfeit drugs, especially those coming from Canada, deserve attention here. In 2007, the international counterfeit drug business was a $30–40 billion industry, and bogus products caused thousands of deaths worldwide. In one instance, only 15 percent of Canadian drugs examined by the FDA actually originated from Canada. In another instance, it was found that 11,000 websites purported to be Canadian – often displaying the maple leaf flag – when in fact there were just 214 Canadian pharmacy websites.[38] While this is troubling, counterfeit pharmaceuticals were a global problem, not exclusively an American and Canadian border concern. They flowed into the US and Canada from all directions, yet the mounting perceived prevalence of counterfeits originating from Canada influenced the Bush administration's policy on drug importation. Based on smaller pilot programs it became clear that the volume of imported, illegal prescription drugs moving into the US was difficult to quantify. Consequently, authorities determined that Canadian drugs constituted a risk to Americans, even though it was tricky to measure that danger.

CONTINUITY AND CHANGE

The Clinton and Bush administrations both opposed the legalization of reimportation. This stance was affirmed in 2000–01, when two successive heads of the Department of Health and Human Services

(HHS) declined to support legislation. In late 2000, passage of the Clinton administration's Medicine Equity and Drug Safety Act would have made it lawful for Americans to buy drugs from sources outside the United States, provided those drugs were originally manufactured in the country. All that was required for the Act to be formalized was the signature of the secretary of HHS – to certify that the safety of the US drug supply could be maintained and costs of drugs reduced. This was not to be.

Secretary Donna Shalala, Clinton's appointment to head HHS, determined such conditions couldn't be reasonably met and decided not to sign the Act. She described the law as disastrously flawed and full of loopholes, citing three reasons for not signing. One, she noted that federal laws required government-approved labelling (FDA) on any prescription drug sold in the country and drug manufacturers could have blocked imports by denying access to the labels. Two, Shalala emphasized that authority for the import program would expire after five years. This meant wholesalers would be reluctant to buy the equipment needed to test and distribute imported drugs since they could not be sure of "long-term financial returns." Last, drug makers had the potential to thwart Congress's intent by requiring distributors to sell their product at high prices. Despite the program's fanfare, support from a number of lobby groups, and her desire to help provide cheaper medications to Americans, Shalala simply killed the drug-import plan. Its flaws, she asserted, "undermine the potential for cost savings associated with prescription drug reimportation and could pose unnecessary public health risks."[39] The demonization of Canadian drugs was just the beginning, and they – as well as their users – were characterized as radical.

Shalala's successor as the head of the Department of Health and Human Services agreed with her. Secretary Tommy Thompson, a Bush appointee, professed a strong belief in the necessity of more affordable drugs, but articulated that he would be sacrificing public safety by essentially opening the closed distribution system. He explained it this way: "Once an FDA-approved prescription drug is exported for sale in another country," he wrote, "it is no longer subject to U.S. requirements and it can no longer be monitored by U.S. regulators."[40] The death of this law not only maintained the closed distribution system, it also demonstrated continuity between the Clinton and Bush administrations and served to crystallize the broader complexity of the reimportation issue. Despite pressure from state and local governments, as well as important political actors, the executive branch refused to be swept up by momentum to reform the closed system.

President Bush nevertheless vacillated on reimportation. In 2000, while running for the highest office in the land, he asserted reimportation "made sense," a view attributed to the fact that Bush did not want to alienate elderly voters in Florida, the largest sector of the population purchasing drugs from Canada. Advocating reimportation of drugs amid a tight election race was certainly very shrewd on Bush's part.[41] Four years later, in the middle of the 2004 presidential campaign, Bush again tacitly supported reimportation, with the caveat that drugs had to be proven safe. His Democratic opponent, John Kerry, challenged the president's position during a live televised debate and accused him of, if not outright lying, then certainly promising one thing while doing another. According to Kerry, Bush had blocked reimportation legislation in 2003; the president, for his part, responded with a reference to the security of the drug supply. Bush defended his obstructionist policy with an argument similar to that made by pharmaceutical companies. It was one that placed Canadian pharmaceuticals in the same category as all sorts of illegal recreational drugs. "When a drug comes in from Canada," Bush countered, "I want to make sure it cures you and doesn't kill you." He continued: "What my worry is, is that, you know, it looks like it's from Canada, and it might be from the third world."[42]

While President Bush adopted a fluid position on reimportation, his appointees at the HHS and FDA did not. In 2002, Tommy Thompson, who had already scuttled the legalization of reimportation, combined US national security imperatives and a policy opposing counterfeit drugs. In his estimation, drugs reimported to the US from Canada constituted a danger to American consumers; building this case, he drew parallels with the new War on Terror launched after September 11, 2001. Thompson warned, "opening our borders to reimported drugs potentially could increase the flow of counterfeit drugs, cheap foreign copies of FDA-approved drugs [what the rest of us call generics], expired and contaminated drugs, and drugs stored under inappropriate and unsafe conditions." Thompson's argument concluded with a reference to the recent terrorist threats in Washington, DC, and around the country: "In light of the anthrax attacks of last fall, that's a risk we simply cannot take."[43]

The Food and Drug Administration supported this position. In fact, FDA commissioner Mark McClellan, President Bush's appointee, became "one of the most loyal soldiers to back the White House on the debate over reimporting drugs from Canada." Under McClellan's leadership, the FDA announced in 2003 that helping others obtain imported drugs could be a civil and criminal offense. In a 12 February 2003 policy letter, McClellan maintained that the FDA could no longer guarantee the safety of such drugs. When McClellan departed, the acting FDA commissioner, Lester Crawford, suggested that terrorists might tamper with prescription drugs imported from Canada and that this was a source of continuing concern. One pharmaceutical industry journalist wrote that Crawford used the "terrorist trump card."[44]

The FDA also took its case to Congress. In fact, one of the agency's senior executives delivered a series of statements before various congressional committees throughout 2001–03. In 2001, Associate Commissioner for Policy, Planning and Legislation William Hubbard testified before the Committee on Commerce, Science, and Transportation. He then gave a similar statement in 2002 to a Senate Special Committee on Aging. During both hearings, Hubbard underscored the importance of vigilance in the fight against the dangers of drug importation. After chronicling the FDA's recent legal struggles with counterfeit criminal enterprises in Alabama, Los Angeles, and Texas, he recounted the gravity of drug importation's risks to public health. "Throwing open the door to drugs purchased by individuals directly from Canadian sellers," Hubbard said of potential legalized importation, "will encourage unscrupulous individuals to devise schemes using Canada as a transshipment point for dangerous products from all around the globe."[45] One implication of this portentous message was that Canadian lawmakers and bureaucrats in Health Canada had to concentrate on the issue of reimportation and tackle the "maple peril."

On 24 June 2003, Hubbard, along with his colleague John M. Taylor, explained the mounting perils of imported drugs. In a presentation titled "A System Overwhelmed: The Avalanche of Imported, Counterfeit and Unapproved Drugs in the U.S.," Hubbard and Taylor traced the agency's ongoing efforts to mitigate that danger. They spoke about the FDA's professional partners, its enforcement activities to date, and drug cost initiatives. In describing the "avalanche," Hubbard and Taylor asserted that the FDA lacked resources to regulate drugs entering the US by mail. In their conclusion, Canada's complicit role in the undermining of the secure, closed system of regulation was again referenced, thereby raising questions about how Canadian officials might address the problem in the future.[46]

The FDA's effort to hinder the avalanche of dangerous drugs included the establishment of a federal Counterfeit Drug Task Force, called Operation Gray Lord. Created in 2003, Gray Lord was administered by the FDA and integrated the DEA, Justice Department, and local law enforcement officials. It was guided by four fundamental principles: (1) preventing the introduction of counterfeit drugs into the American market; (2) facilitating the identification of counterfeit drugs; (3) minimising the risk and exposure of consumers to counterfeit drugs; and (4) avoiding the addition of unnecessary costs on the prescription drug distribution system.

According to McClellan, "[d]ifferent kinds of drug imports carry different risks," and the task force, whose name befitted a James Bond novel, was intended to minimize those risks. Adding even more of a cloak-and-dagger aspect to the story, one task force interim report proposed the use of several cutting-edge security technologies to safeguard the US drug supply and stave off counterfeits. These technologies were of both overt and covert natures and included radio frequency identification, micro-barcode tags, organic tags, optically variable devices, laser perforations, and digital watermarks. The Task Force suggested the use of such technologies so regulators and consumers could better authenticate, verify, and track legitimate and illegitimate drug products.[47]

PROPAGATING FEAR, CREATING DOUBT

As Health and Human Services and Food and Drug Administration officials weighed in on the threats posed by Canadian pharmaceuticals, other parties in the medical marketplace sought to sway the contested legalization of reimportation practices. The Pharmaceutical Research and Manufacturers Association (PhRMA), a trade association and lobby group, for example, clearly wanted to curb drugs imported to the US from Canada, especially as Medicare prescription drug coverage (the MMA) was being debated on Capitol Hill. First, PhRMA earmarked over $1 million "to change the Canadian health care system" and "another $450,000 to prevent Canadian internet-pharmacies from selling low-price drugs to U.S. customers." The exact meaning of "change" remained unclear. In addition, PhRMA was actively lobbying Congress to adopt market-based solutions to rising drug costs rather than easing restrictions on drugs coming from outside the US. Reimportation, from the drug industry's perspective, was not an appropriate solution. After the 2002 congressional elections, the drug industry spent a record $91.4 million on federal lobbying activities, not including the $50 million used to influence Congress through advertising, direct mail, telemarketing, and grants to advocacy groups.[48]

The effort was aimed at fomenting fear and doubt about reimportation and, ultimately, radicalizing Canadian pharmaceuticals. In 2003, such major pharmaceutical companies as AstraZeneca, GlaxoSmithKline, Pfizer, and Wyeth used the pretext of safety and security to pressure both Canadian and American authorities to limit cross-border purchasing. In early 2003, GlaxoSmithKline (GSK) threatened to stop supplying some Canadian pharmacies. The Anglo-American pharmaceuticals group wrote to Canadian retailers and wholesalers and warned them it would take action if they continued selling prescription drugs to US customers. In February 2004, Pfizer cut off two Canadian wholesalers. *Fortune* reported, "it was the most dramatic and resounding escalation to date in the raging war between the pharmaceutical industry and American seniors over the illicit practice of importing cheap prescription drugs from Canada."[49]

Another tactic was to direct advertisements at consumers. One particular ad, sponsored by the drug industry, depicted two identical-looking pills over the caption *Quick. Pick the Capsule that Hasn't Been Tampered With*. The advertisement cited the support not just of the FDA and HHS, but the US Customs Service and Border Patrol and the DEA, arms of government usually concerned with protecting Americans from illicit drugs. The ad warned, furthermore, that allowing Americans to fill prescriptions in Canada "could open America's medicine cabinets to an influx of dangerous drugs," and closed with an appeal to "Keep Black Market Drugs Out of America."[50] Ominous government advertisements also influenced Americans not to purchase drugs from Canada. A poster sponsored by the FDA and CBP also cast doubts on the safety and quality of foreign drugs. Reading, "Buying Medicine from Outside the U.S. Is Risky Business," this ad featured a vicious green snake, with fangs bared and piercing golden eyes, squeezing a bottle of pills. To the right of the viper, the ad asked Americans: "Think it's safe buying medicine from outside the United States? Think again." If nothing else, the image was reminiscent of Just Say No posters and public service announcements about what the brain looks like on drugs.

In due course, the research and strategy behind the advertising campaign surfaced. Through industrious reporting by the *Wall Street Journal* it was revealed how PhRMA, the same organization lobbying Congress and seeking to change Canada's healthcare system, had hired a prestigious public relations firm, Edelman, to develop a communication campaign to halt cross-border drug reimportation. Edelman's associates discovered after conducting market research and focus group tests that the issue of illegality failed to register with American consumers; instead, "fear and accountability" shifted American consumer perceptions about drugs from places such as Canada and Mexico. Edelman subsequently advised PhRMA to craft advertisements that fomented suspicions about the safety and effectiveness of drugs bought from foreign sources.[51] Edelman, that is, advised drug companies to exploit fear for their advantage.

The Canadian reaction to American policy was fundamentally, and in a stereotypically Canadian way, accommodating. Canadian government officials were clearly aware of potential pitfalls inherent in cross-border drug purchasing. In May 2003, Canada's deputy minister of health, Diane Gorman, emphasized Canada could not vouch for the safety of drugs exported to the United States. In June 2003, Health Canada released a paper that warned Canadians and Americans about the risks associated with Internet pharmacies. "If you buy drugs on line," the document stated, "you may be putting your health at serious risk."[52] Canadian alignment with American policy was further highlighted in 2006 when the Criminal Intelligence Service Canada (CISC) published a policy paper on counterfeit drugs in western industrialized countries. According to the CISC, the counterfeit pharmaceuticals trade in China, Southeast Asia, and Africa was endemic. Nevertheless, it was also a burgeoning phenomenon in Canada and the US, countries with advanced and formidable systems of regulation, control, and enforcement. The 2006 CISC document reaffirmed Hubbard's testimony from years past and pointed to several US-led law enforcement projects demonstrating how organized counterfeit pharmaceutical operations trafficked multiple types of controlled medications simultaneously. What's more, the article acknowledged, "new, expensive medicines such as hormones, corticosteroids, cancer drugs or antivirals are the most frequently counterfeited medications in industrialized countries."[53]

Canadian pharmaceutical and health officials were also quick to denounce the practice of reimportation and to support American regulators and the pharmaceutical industry. By 2003, the Canadian Medical Association (CMA), the Canadian Pharmacists Association (cPhA), and the Canadian Association of Retail Pharmacy Regulatory Authorities (CARPRA) all publicly opposed the practice. This opposition took three forms. First, on 22 April 2003, the CMA advocated support of tighter limitations because, under the Canadian Code of Ethics, physicians had a responsibility to conduct a patient history and examination and thereafter to discuss the benefits and risks of a given drug. This often does not occur when drugs are purchased via the internet. Second, on 13 May 2003, the cPhA endorsed the restriction on the illegal importation of prescription drugs. Third, Canada's pharmacy regulatory body, CARPRA, made a joint statement with its American equivalent, the National Association of Boards of Pharmacy (NABP), calling on law enforcement agencies to promote compliance with federal, state, and provincial pharmacy laws and standards. This joint statement, announced 7 May, was the first of its kind and represented a mutual aversion to the growing trend of drug reimportation. Canadian and American authorities equally recognized the dangers of reimportation and sought to stifle the flow of Canadian drugs southward.

BACKLASH

Despite condemnation of reimportation by both American and Canadian regulatory officials, this position was far from unanimous and indeed the debate about drug reimportation was stirring. For example, Tim Pawlenty, the governor of Minnesota, a front-runner for vice-president on the Republican ticket in 2008, actively promoted cross-border purchasing. He disdainfully called FDA warning letters "snotty-grams." Similarly, Dr Alastair Wood, whose nomination for FDA commissioner had been blocked by drug companies, suggested McClellan's policies were flawed. "I'm less impressed with the danger of Canadian drugs than Mark [McClellan] appears to be. It's hard for me to believe that Pfizer is selling drugs that are less safe in Canada."[54]

One raucous congressional hearing saw members of the House Subcommittee on Human Rights and Wellness proclaim that the FDA was playing politics with American lives and ought to allow importation of drugs from Canada. High drug prices were a bipartisan issue, and both Democratic and Republican lawmakers lambasted the FDA, arguing that the agency possessed no evidence of either a security or safety problem with Canadian drugs. Its warnings were tantamount to fear-mongering propaganda. "You scare the hell out of them," said Representative Dan Burton (R-IN), chair of the subcommittee. Representative Bernie Sanders (I-VT), who made significant waves during the 2016 Democratic primaries, also weighed in. "You should be putting out pamphlets saying people have been going across the border ... and there hasn't been one problem," he scolded. In essence, Burton and Sanders charged that the FDA shifted its policy because of drug industry pressure. In reference to the drug reimportation bill he sponsored in 2003, Gil Gutknecht (R-MN) asserted that the FDA was attempting "to undermine a legislative initiative the American people desperately want and need."[55]

The US Senate also addressed the issue of the safety and security of reimported drugs. Senator Byron Dorgan (D-ND) placed a formal hold on Mark McClellan's nomination as head of Medicare and Medicaid. Motivating Dorgan's move was the fact that McClellan had not appeared before the panel to discuss drug imports as he was asked to do. Dorgan, who supported importation legislation during the Clinton years, found that his political manoeuvre worked. McClellan testified before the Senate Commerce Committee, chaired by Senator John McCain, and the potential FDA chief was rewarded with scornful criticism. During the proceedings, members of the Commerce Committee attacked the FDA's views and tactics and pressed McClellan to come up with a plan for allowing safe imports. McClellan dodged. He referred back to the security issue, noting, "we want to be flexible in working with Congress to address these safety concerns." He added that the FDA did not have a "specific proposal" for legalized importation and stated cagily that it was not within his purview. McCain, an ostensible expert in national security issues, responded: "We rely on the administration and people like you to give us proposals so we can examine them ... I think it's time the administration came up with a proposal."[56]

Apart from the political hostility in Washington, DC, everyday Americans were mostly in favour of access to cheaper drugs, regardless of safety issues. An October 2003 *Wall Street Journal / Harris Interactive* poll demonstrated widespread support for cheaper drugs, even illegal ones. The poll found that 77 percent of Americans surveyed thought it unreasonable for pharmaceutical companies to prevent Canadian internet pharmacies from selling their drugs to Americans. Stony Brook University carried out its own national survey and found that 58 percent of American consumers felt Canadian drugs were safe or somewhat safe. A further 68 percent of respondents felt that reimportation ought to be legalized. Moreover, the Kaiser Family Foundation conducted similar polls and revealed that a majority of consumers by and large supported drug reimportation and initiatives easing access to Canadian drugs.[57]

Political activity at the state level also indicated support for access to Canadian pharmaceutical products. Between 2002 and September 2005, both Republicans and Democrats proposed over 190 bills in multiple state legislatures which would have eased restrictions on reimportation or would have facilitated the purchase of pharmaceuticals from Canada. Additionally, the number of attempts to pass legislation at the federal and state level accelerated from three per year in 2002 to eighty-four per year by September 2005. For example, the mayor of Springfield, MA, made national headlines when he encouraged the importation of pharmaceuticals from Canada for city employees and retirees. In 2003, Governor Rod Blagojevich (D-IL), who was later forced to resign due to various criminal charges, announced, "we're not to violate what the FDA's rules are, but we are going to try and get the FDA to change its position ... the FDA cannot ignore the people forever."[58]

AFTERMATH

Between 2000 and 2005, cheaper drugs reimported from Canada to the United States undoubtedly saved Americans money and generated substantial disputation. The debate about this cross-border trade traversed traditional party lines and prompted local, state, and national legislative initiatives on an increasing scale. It was a debate complicated by the absence of reliable data and hard evidence from the border between Canada and the US – just like various other cases in this book. For example, the unconvincing science surrounding heroin in palliative care settings proved divisive, just as it was with Laetrile and LSD. These drugs occupied intermediate spaces. They remained subjects of debate, considered both magic bullets and dangerous drugs, depending on the person. It was the same, then, with a whole swath of pharmaceutical products in the wake of September 11. At stake, though, was not the individual choice about *one* specific pharmaceutical product, but the safety of multiple products from Canada. Meanwhile, public opinion poll results tended to favour access and affordability over safety. At any rate, many Americans' beliefs aligned with Alastair Wood's: it was simply too hard to fathom that Pfizer, or any major pharmaceutical company, would sell inferior drugs in Canada. Also, the story of reimportation and "the maple peril" underlines that scare tactics aren't just used in the realm of illicit drugs. Public service announcements have warned against crack cocaine, with brains as eggs fried on skillets. Anslinger carefully crafted a linkage between madness, crime, degeneracy, and cannabis. These are well-known historical examples. Yet, it's worthwhile to unpack how legitimate pharmaceutical products have been characterized. The preceding discussion embodied many of the core themes in this book: the economics and evidence behind medicine and health policy, medical tourism, and the various paths a drug may take.

What is clear is that, yes, the security of the American drug supply was indeed compromised by reimportation. In measured tones, William Hubbard of the FDA described how regulators could not possibly verify the safety of pharmaceuticals entering the United States from anywhere else, including Canada. In short, this burgeoning trade in pharmaceuticals undermined and penetrated the protective shield that was the American closed distribution system, a point of pride for Big Pharma, law enforcement agencies, and the FDA. At the same time, the dangers of reimportation were surely exaggerated – that is, Canadian drugs were demonized and radicalized – to deter American consumers from purchasing cheaper pharmaceuticals and lend legitimacy to HHS, FDA, and CBP policies. Good drugs had become bad news. This came in the form of political rhetoric, advertisements, and policies, many of which might have been aimed at illicit drugs. The next chapter of this book will narrow its focus to explore obesity and how certain diet pills changed career paths.

AMERICAN OBESITY AND DIET PILLS: DANGEROUS DRUGS ON EVERY CORNER

In *The Wonderful Wizard of Oz*, by L. Frank Baum, all of the characters were in search of something. Dorothy was looking for a way home. The Scarecrow needed a brain, whereas the Tin Man sought a heart and the Lion wanted courage. The only way to attain their goals – to find what they were looking for – was to visit the Wizard of Oz in the Emerald City. His magic would grant their wishes. The wizard turned out to be a fraud, however. He was a charlatan, just an ordinary man trying to protect his position and empire. In 2014, life imitated art. TV's Dr Oz was given a public lashing for his promotion of spurious weight-loss products when called before a Senate committee on consumer protection.

In front of the cameras and captured by C-SPAN, Oz admitted he was a bit of a cheerleader, using flowery language to promote certain brands, although he also suggested that it was important to advertise multiple views on the show. The reaction was swift and merciless. John Oliver, of *Last Week Tonight*, came down hard on Oz. He taunted and belittled the TV doctor. He used all the bells and whistles he could, including actor Steve Buscemi, to continue the public lashing. Likewise, *New York Times* columnist Frank Bruni described Oz as having "morphed not just willingly but exuberantly into a carnival barker" and "a one-man morality play about the temptations of mammon and the seduction of applause." Then, a group of ten high-profile doctors called for the removal of Oz in a public letter. They argued that he was pushing "miracle" weight-loss supplements with no scientific proof that they worked. Oz had displayed an "egregious lack of integrity," said the letter, and had shown "disdain for science and for evidence-based medicine." It suggested that he had "misled and endangered" the public with this approach.[1]

Part bluster, part public relations, the letter was not entirely off-base. It was certainly true about green coffee, which was just one of the products Dr Oz promoted. Green coffee refers to a dietary supplement called Pure Green Coffee, whose manufacturers have claimed stunningly high weight-loss possibilities. The Federal Trade Commission disagreed. The Commission sued the makers of Pure Green Coffee, accusing them of making bogus claims and tricking vulnerable American consumers. The drugs, the FTC says, are ineffective. Yet, Oz – a cardiothoracic surgeon – took none of this lying down. In late April, he came back at his critics, including the doctors who had penned the damning letter. In a frisky defence of himself, Oz restated his conviction that consumers should know whether the food at their stores originates from genetically modified organisms. As for the letter, Oz characterized it as a smear intended to shut him up and vowed: "We will not be silenced." In a sop to his supporters, he claimed that the biotech industry and makers of GMOs – big business – were behind the ad hominem attack on him.[2]

Controversies like the one that surrounded Dr Oz's promotion of weight loss cures are not entirely new. The author-promoters of diet sensations in the 1970s and 1980s – or Oz, for that matter – do not represent a fresh trend in American culture. Rather, Atkins and Oz are part of a long and extravagant procession of diet experts who lived well and got rich while dispensing weight-loss wisdom. In short, since the late nineteenth century, American doctors, tycoons, and outright hustlers all added to a distinct dieting discourse that intersected with conceptions of body image, social behaviour, and market imperatives. For more than a century, American consumers have sought safe and effective ways to drop pounds, tighten up, and slim down, and, as a nation, it has been a losing battle. The books haven't worked, and neither have all the drugs. According to the biologist and historian Roberta J. Park, obesity and fitness have featured in American thought and writings since at least 1879.[3] Yet, the number of people who are overweight or obese has reached epidemic proportions, with authorities estimating that 61 percent of US adults fall into one of those categories. This means that obesity – depending on the year – constitutes one of the leading causes of preventable death, after smoking. Now, though, we are living in the era of surgery as well as the *Fattening of America* and as a consequence a nascent *Fat Politics*.[4]

Beauty and attractiveness are, of course, complicated ideas. On the one hand, *fashionable beauty* may be regarded as a short-term concept driven by a media/fashion/entertainment nexus for multiple underlying reasons. *Physical attraction*, on the other hand, remains a hardwired biological concept undergirded by objective research studies. While there is no consensus and the lines are certainly murky, the literature suggests that hip-to-waist ratios, for instance, may be evolutionary and cross-cultural.[5] If nothing else, the evolutionary foundation for objective beauty standards bolsters the need to examine the perpetual diet crazes.

Fashion and acceptable levels of weight are, then, fluid conceptions shaped by companies such as Green Coffee and Dr Oz, as well as government food guidelines, magazines, and movies. Surely beauty, as measured by the senses, is subjective by definition. Upon seeing a beautiful person or a beautiful piece of art and commenting, "wow, beautiful," we are typically referring to the superficial sensation of beauty afforded by the interplay of light and shadow and colour or underlying patterns and symmetry. At one point in time, corpulence was a sign of power and affluence. It indicated wealth. Busty, full-figured women – in the Marilyn Monroe mold – were *de rigueur*. When *Sports Illustrated*, *Maxim*, *Elle*, and *Cosmopolitan* showcased Ashley Graham, a plus-size model, on the cover of their magazines, this undoubtedly reflected and altered perceptions of beauty in American society. When Kesha shot back at "body-shaming" bullies on social media, her reaction undoubtedly influenced people's views of body issues.[6]

Even as ideal weights and proportions have shifted – think Monroe and Twiggy, Moss and Kardashian – popular weight-loss methods have done the same. Some of the treatments have included prescription and over-the-counter drugs and dietary supplements, as well as surgical procedures such as gastro-intestinal bypass surgery, gastroplasty (stomach stapling), and jaw wiring. Other methods have included the television shows of motivational weight-loss gurus; commercial weight-loss centres; commercial diet drinks; doctor-supervised very-low-calorie diets, complete with their own vitamin shots, fibre cookies, and drinks; the development of fat-free, low-fat, fake-fat, and sugar-free foods; weight-loss support groups; exercise trends such as aerobics and body building; and cellulite creams. This list, while not even close to comprehensive, offers a window into the breadth of available products. In short, there are lots to choose from. As Americans have sought to modify their bodies, the historical record illustrates that it's best to be wary of false wizards like Dr Oz. This chapter will showcase how diet pills were scrutinized in the late 1970s and 1980s, at a time when Laetrile caught the public's attention and medical heroin also forced conversations. And it will conclude in 2001, when cross-border pharmaceutical purchasing grew into a hot-button political issue.

TRAGEDY

On 6 June 1978, Gloria Jean Davis's head began throbbing. Stars danced and flashed in her field of vision, she collapsed, and then her right arm and leg became partly paralyzed. An active twenty-six-year-old Florida native who often took Appedrine, a non-prescription diet pill made by Thompson Medical Company, Gloria had no history of hypertension, and when she sued Thompson she was awarded an out-of-court settlement of $125,000. One of the company's representatives stated that Thompson settled the suit simply to avoid expensive litigation.[7] A more recent example of the dangers of diet pills for American citizens is Tricia Newenham, from Maine. In 2000, Tricia, who took cough and cold medicines and the occasional appetite suppressant, suffered a hemorrhagic stroke. She spent a month in a coma, and thereafter emerged totally blind and mentally impaired. According to a poignant *Los Angeles Times* article, Tricia, fifteen at the time of her stroke, was preparing for college, the first in her family to do so, and was a recreational swimmer and softball player. Tricia's parents, a nurse and a plumber, were nearly bankrupted by the resulting hospital bills, but a settlement with a major drug company, Novartis, eased their financial burden. When first alerted to the connection between diet pills with phenylpropanolamine (PPA) and strokes, Tricia's stepfather was puzzled and angry. "It never even dawned on us. It was in the store. Everyone uses it. It must be all right."[8]

Tricia's stepfather was not the only bewildered American citizen. In the late 1970s, the safety of PPA, an essential ingredient in over-the-counter diet aids as well as cold and cough medicines, began to be disputed by Congress, the US Food and Drug Administration (FDA), and health watchdog organizations. Researchers, doctors, health advocates, and regulators demonstrated division about the safety and effectiveness of such diet pills. While PPA was extremely popular and likely a part of the average American's medicine cabinet, members of the US House of Representatives and activists in the Center for Science in the Public Interest charged that it was linked to strokes, hypertension, potentially fatal heart problems, kidney disease, and muscle damage.[9] Meanwhile, critics also charged that such weight loss drugs as Appedrine, Acutrim, and Dexatrim were scarcely even effective.

By the time of Gloria Jean's and Tricia's tragedies, American consumers had already long searched for safe and effective approaches to losing weight. "Weight loss gizmos and potions have been in existence since the 1800s," but the post-war period saw an explosion in the diet industry.[10] According to *Time* magazine, this was paradoxical, since "the U.S. is one of the fattest countries on earth, and at the same time the most obsessed with slimness."[11] With Hillel Schwartz's *Never Satisfied* and Peter Stearns's *Fat History*, which stretch back to the nineteenth century, we have moved into the realm of cultural analysis. In Stearns's view, "dieting, weight consciousness, and widespread hostility to obesity form one of the fundamental themes in modern life" in the United States.[12] Diet pills and dieting more generally are without doubt a mass cultural phenomenon, and through a more sophisticated understanding of one drug technology in this saga, we should be able to enhance our perspectives on health, gender, and "fatness" in the twentieth century.[13]

BANTING, BEYONCÉ, AND THE BEAUTIFUL BODY

The author-promoters of diet sensations in the 1970s and 1980s were far from novel. In 1863, British doctor William Banting was the first to produce a bestselling diet book, *A Letter on Corpulence*, which went through twelve editions by 1900 and sold extremely well in the United States. Thereafter, Horace Fletcher's *AB-Z of Our Own Nutrition*, one of his many books, created a cultural sensation with its emphasis on excessive chewing. Fletcher was known as the "Great Masticator," and his distinguished appearance, feats of strength at a relatively advanced age, and high-profile acolytes made him a public personality in the mid-1890s. Sporting a dandy white suit (much like Tom Wolfe) and a cane, Fletcher pushed easy-to-remember messages, including "nature will castigate those who don't masticate," and boasted about transforming "a pitiable glutton into an intelligent epicurean." Just be sure to chew your food over a hundred times, he said, and with the support of individuals such as John D. Rockefeller and Upton Sinclair, "Fletcherizing" grabbed the public's attention. For author Michael Pollan, Fletcher was one of the country's first diet gurus.[14]

The year Fletcher died, 1919, witnessed the entry of women into the diet book market.[15] Dr Lulu Peters, a graduate of the University of California, Berkeley's medical school, syndicated columnist, and one-time overweight woman, published *Diet and Health: With Key to the Calories* during 1918–19, which immediately found a wide readership. At the time of the book's release, Peters was stationed in Bosnia while working with the Red Cross. Eventually selling over 2 million copies, the "witty and whimsical" book not only introduced calorie counting (advocating 1,200 maximum) to America's weight-conscious citizens, it did so using humour and the rhetoric of self-determination, self-discipline, and empowerment. On the one hand, she suggested that dieting represented patriotism amid World War One. Corsets – mandated by the War Industries Board – were sacrificed for the war effort. Peters suggested that "for every pang of hunger we feel we can have a double joy, that of knowing we are saving worse pangs in some little children, and that of knowing that for every pang we feel we lose a pound." She also recommended that women organize Watch Your Weight Anti-Kaiser Classes to obtain it. On the other hand, Peters was a suffragist, and in the age of the "flapper" and the 19th Amendment to the US Constitution, she couched her book in the language of health for the "New Woman" and self-sufficiency.[16]

Lulu Hunt Peters (1873–1930) was born in Maine but moved to California in her youth. She was always overweight, and when she didn't outgrow her baby fat as she had hoped, she set about researching a problem that was so personal to her. After earning her medical degree, she began devising a solution to the problem of being overweight. Through a sensible regimen of calorie-counting and self-control, Peters lost 32 kilograms and began a public-health campaign to educate women about healthy diet, exercise, and weight loss. Her bestselling book remained in the top ten non-fiction bestselling books from 1922 to 1926 and was accessible to a wide audience, often recounting personal anecdotes from fictional characters such as Ima Gobbler, Natty B. Slymm, and Tiny Weyaton. More importantly, it showed women how to calculate their ideal weight with a formula. Her book included estimates of food portions that would contain 100 calories, based on research in a variety of technical publications that were not available to the general reader. She also indicated how many calories someone should eat per pound of ideal body weight, to keep the ideal weight that her system suggests (similar to the Body Mass Index). To achieve the ideal body, in other words, you had to crunch numbers and count calories. In addition, the *Master Cleanse* diet emerged in the mid-1940s and was thereafter formally published by Stanley Burroughs in the mid-1970s. Essentially a ten-day fast, the plan allowed for lemon juice, cayenne pepper, maple syrup, and water, and it has seen a resurgence in recent times, with Beyoncé, Jared Leto, Demi Moore, and Ashton Kutcher all publicly praising the plan.

While "the portion of middle-aged Americans who are clinically obese has doubled since the 1960s," the number who are "grossly overweight" has increased 350 percent over the past thirty years.[17] At the turn of the twenty-first century, being overweight and obesity constituted the second leading cause of preventable death in the United States (after smoking) and an estimated 300,000 deaths per year were the result. In dollar terms, the cost of this struggle exceeded $100 billion per year. In 2001, nearly 29 percent of men and 44 percent of women (or 68 million American adults) were trying to lose weight. According to one estimate in 2000, consumers spent $34.7 billion on weight-loss products and programs.[18] Even as this "obesity epidemic" grew more pronounced over the past forty years, a "national health and fitness movement" gripped the United States in the 1970s and 1980s.[19] In fact, the issue became so critical to Americans' well-being that the federal government took an active role in establishing terms of reference and guidelines. In 1974, for example, the Senate Select Committee on Nutrition and Human Needs held hearings on a national nutrition policy study.[20] Two years later, the same committee published the unequivocally titled report *Diet Related to Killer Diseases*. Compelling and candid, the report highlighted the linkage between diets high in fat with heart disease and cholesterol, and those high in sodium and low in fibre with heart disease and certain types of cancer. The next year, in 1977, the Senate published its *Dietary Goals for the United States*, which identified a "target and healthy" diet for Americans and underlined the value of eating foods in their natural and unprocessed state.[21] Then, in 1980, the inaugural set of "Dietary Guidelines for Americans" was established by the

Department of Health and Human Services and the US Department of Agriculture.[22] Ever since, a new set has appeared every five years. By the end of the 1980s, moreover, two major reports, the 1988 *Surgeon General's Report on Nutrition and Health* and the National Academy of Sciences' 1989 report *Diet and Health: Implications for Reducing Chronic Disease*, pointed to the critical role of diet and lifestyle in maintaining health.[23]

Meanwhile, as the US Senate, the executive branch, and the National Academy of Sciences presented research and guidelines, Americans demonstrated an increased interest in the pursuit of weight loss and fitness. In attempting to capture the moment, historian Robert M. Collins described this development as part of a new, postmodern "therapeutic culture" wherein Americans, both men and women, sought to improve the quality of their lives and individual satisfaction.[24] Millions of dollars were spent on Jane Fonda exercise videotapes, health club memberships, low-calorie foods, and other means of attaining a trim figure. In 1987, health clubs grossed $5 billion, diet foods $74 billion, and vitamin products $2.7 billion. Diet plans and diet books that emphasized a variety of spurious approaches, ranging from low fat to low carbohydrate, to a focus on cabbage soup, to, more extreme, the ingestion of tapeworms, exploded in popularity. By 1984, according to Hillel Schwartz, the market was saturated with over 300 different diet books, to say nothing of the ubiquity of diet-related articles in such popular magazines as *Self*, *Prevention*, and *American Health*.[25] According to one account, at least twenty-four diet books achieved bestseller status by 1987, with titles like *Fit for Life* and *The Beverley Hills Diet*. Although the approach to weight loss diverged in the numerous books available, the ubiquity of the books themselves suggests a particular preoccupation with the "beautiful body."[26] It is in the core concepts of such books – self-control, self-perfection, and perfectability – that one can discern how American cultural impulses construct versions of women and bodies, and why new technologies are needed to achieve these bodies.

Throughout the 1980s, exercise videos appeared on weekly *Billboard* lists of the ten top-selling home video products.[27] For

---

* Rees argues that American consumers in the 1980s increasingly recognized the value of informed choice and the explosive growth of popular health literature was a response to the public's voracious appetite for health information.

instance, Jane Fonda was undoubtedly the pioneer and inspirational superstar that connected commercial beauty culture and the body culture of health and fitness. Using the rhetoric of empowerment, she was "able to credibly link the discourse of health with that of beauty" and a growing concern of the baby-boom generation about aging. In doing so, she influenced a raft of stars, including David Carradine, Lou Ferrigno, Martina Navratilova, Debbie Reynolds, Arnold Schwarzenegger, and Raquel Welch, to make videos that would sell over 15 million copies by the end of the 1980s.[28] (In Canada, of course, Hal Johnson and Joanne McLeod's "BodyBreaks" were ubiquitous on the television.)

Multiple positive messages coursed through these videos and, more broadly, underpinned Americans' vast expenditures on the goods and services aimed at reducing their weight. According to *Better Homes and Gardens* in 1984, "Telling Americans how to lose weight definitely is big business."[29] Advertisements for diet pills and supplements have routinely employed the same slogans and themes to increase sales: rapid weight loss (users could lose 8 to 10 pounds per week), consumer testimonials and before/after photos ("I lost 55 lbs in 30 days"), long-term and permanent weight loss claims ("take it off and keep it off"), and no diet or exercise required ("you can eat as much as you want and still lose weight") were and remain the techniques dominating the marketing of weight loss products. Just as important, advertisements regularly highlighted that supplements or pills were "clinically proved and doctor approved."[30] A final message often conveyed in weight-loss ads pertained to the inherent naturalness and safety of the product.

Irrespective of the success or failure of one particular advertising message, over the past hundred years or so Americans have turned to numerous weight-loss drugs and remedies to solve their problems. Some medications were legitimate, while others were specious and perilous. In the early 1900s, popular weight-loss drugs included animal-derived thyroid, laxatives, and arsenic and strychnine. On occasion, doctors in the 1930s prescribed dinitrophenol (DNP), a synthetic insecticide and herbicide that increased human metabolism so dramatically that it caused organs to fail. By the 1950s, human chorionic gonadotropin (HCG) grew more popular, though the FDA later exposed it as ineffective. In the 1970s, people would go so far as to ingest beef tapeworms, which could afterward be eradicated with antibiotics. In addition, with the passage of the Dietary Supplement

Popular diet plans of the 1980s and 1990s

Name	Company/ founder	1st year on US market	Book	Focus
Dr Atkins' Diet Revolution	Dr Robert Atkins	1972	*Dr. Atkins' Diet Revolution* (1972)	Low carbohydrate intake
California Diet	Dr Peter Wood	1983	*California Diet and Exercise Program* (1983)	Extreme caloric intake reduction
Cambridge Diet	Dr Allan Howard	1980	No book	Meal replacement and nitrogen balance
The Carbohydrate Craver's Diet	Dr Judith Wurtman	1982	*The Carbohydrate Craver's Diet* (1982)	Low carbohydrate intake
Diet Center Inc.	Sybil Ferguson	1969; 1st franchise in 1973	*The Diet Center Cookbook* (1986)	Individualized program and meal replacement
The F-Plan Diet	Audrey Eyton	1983	*The F-Plan Diet* (1987) and *F2 Diet* (2007)	Increased intake of dietary fibre
The Pritikin Permanent Weight-Loss Manual	Nathan Pritikin	1979	*The Pritikin Program for Diet and Exercise* (1979) and *The Pritikin Permanent Weight-loss Manual* (1981)	Naturalism; whole and raw foods
The Complete Scarsdale Medical Diet	Dr Herman Tarnower	1978	*The Complete Scarsdale Diet Plus Dr. Tarnower's Lifetime Keep-Slim Program* (1978)	Extreme caloric intake reduction
Shaklee Slim Plan	Dr Forrest C. Shaklee	1956	No book	Meal replacement and metabolism boosting
Weight Watchers	Jean Nidetch	1963	*The Memoir of a Successful Loser: The Story of Weight Watchers* (1972)	Science-based approach to create "calorie deficit"

Health and Education Act in 1994, the United States consumer saw an explosion in dietary supplement marketing, as the law mandated that dietary supplements did not require FDA approval before going to the market and the FDA could only restrict usage or prohibit their sale if they proved to be dangerous. As a result, many supplements in the American marketplace have little value, and some are even associated with serious risks.[31] In recent years, methods of weight loss have begun to include more and more radical options. Surgical procedures such as gastro-intestinal bypass, gastroplasty (stomach stapling), liposuctions, and jaw wiring are just a few examples of what Jonathan Rowe and Judith Silverstein call "one growth sector with a bright future."[32]

The United States Food and Drug Administration, the regulatory agency responsible for diet pills, was certainly aware of the hazards associated with weight-loss solutions. According to the *New York Times* in the mid-1980s, Americans had "an obsession with trim waistlines" and "the chance to make dollars off diets has attracted a remarkable assortment of businesses."[33] While the FDA delayed action with diet pills, the agency demonstrated aggressiveness with other diet products. In 1982, after receiving numerous adverse reaction reports about "starch blockers" – including vomiting, stomach pains, and diarrhea – the FDA tested and declared them illegal. It then moved swiftly to seize over one million tablets.[34] By 1984–85, the FDA also began to attack fraudulent weight-reducing aids. "There's always someone one step ahead of us dreaming up the next crazy thing to knock off pounds," said one FDA official, but the agency sought to keep pace. In testing hundreds of diet pills during the mid-1980s, drug officials occasionally discovered disturbing ingredients: in one instance, dried cow brains. Lastly, the agency investigated the safety of such devices as body wraps, electrical muscle stimulators, and sauna suits that purportedly helped customers lose weight through dehydration or circulatory constriction.[35] For Dennis Myers, the head of the FDA's over-the-counter drug office in the mid-1980s, this invariably led to unscrupulous practices. "There are always people out there trying to make a buck out of fraudulent diet products. It's a continuing problem."[36]

In the 1990s, drugs remained just as important in repurposing the flabby bodies in the United States. A 1992 National Institutes of Health (NIH) panel concluded that approximately one-third of the US population was considered overweight. Using the Body Mass Index (BMI), which is calculated by dividing one's weight in kilograms by height in metres squared, the panel linked obesity to various health risks, including cancer, cardiovascular disease, diabetes, high cholesterol, hypertension, and sleep deprivation. In 1994, an Institute of Medicine study stated that obesity ought to be regarded as a chronic condition like hypertension, not just a problem of will power. The study also found that 30 million Americans were obese and proposed that physicians should treat obesity with drug therapy or with surgery.

In 1994–96, the Fen-Phen combination was increasingly prescribed and accepted in American society. Major newspapers and magazines, such as *Allure, Reader's Digest*, and *Time*, promoted the new weight-loss cocktail. More than 6 million prescriptions were written for the diet combination before it was withdrawn. Sales for Pondimin and Redux reached $300 million, and $1 billion in sales were projected for the future. This was accomplished even though the FDA did not review the studies that examined the Fen-Phen combination or issue an approval for its use. At the same time, from 1994 to 1997, the FDA reviewed over 800 reports of adverse effects associated with Fen-Phen.

In July 1997, new findings on the safety of Fen-Phen treatments created a controversy when Dr Heidi Connelly of the Mayo Clinic revealed her experience treating women with heart problems. The findings, reported in the *New England Journal of Medicine*, suggested that fenfluramine and dexfenfluramine were the likely cause of pulmonary hypertension (also known as primary pulmonary hypertension) and heart valve abnormalities. It was also found that over a quarter of patients who were evaluated demonstrated abnormal echocardiograms. Both Pondimin and Redux were voluntarily withdrawn from the market on 15 September 1997.

Two years after the withdrawal of Fen-Phen, over 11,000 plaintiffs filed over 6,500 lawsuits. Some of the suits focused on heart valve damage, while others focused on primary pulmonary hypertension. Wyeth then established a $3.75 billion national settlement program in 2000, a fund that was later supplemented with another $1.3 billion in 2004. In September 2012, Pfizer, which had purchased Wyeth, lost a court challenge to have claims against Fen-Phen dismissed. The judge ruled that there was enough scientific evidence to demonstrate that PPH, as well as Pulmonary Arterial Hypertension, had significant latency periods. This meant that an individual could be diagnosed many years after taking the drug and could thereby launch further lawsuits.

Phenylpropanolamine (PPA) was one of many accepted tools and techniques used to correct obesity in the last century. Closely related to the phenethylamine and amphetamine classes of drugs, PPA was employed as a stimulant, decongestant, and anorectic agent. Used in products that were virtually ubiquitous, PPA was available in most medicine cabinets: Appedrine, Acutrim, Dexatrim, Dimetapp, and Triaminic are just a few examples. A non-methylated form of ephedrine, PPA was synthesized as early as 1910. Initially called norepinephrine, a patent for it was filed in 1921, while the first human pharmacological studies using the drug were performed ten years later in France. PPA's ability to provoke weight loss in humans was first discovered in 1939 by Dr L.S. Hirsh, a Cleveland-based physician, and subsequent research conducted on rats at New York University, Princeton, and the University of Pennsylvania found that PPA acted on the hypothalamus, the brain's appetite centre.[*37]

Throughout most of its history, phenylpropanolamine has been available over the counter, yet this position has been contested a number of times. In 1957, a federal Committee on Government Operations conducted hearings regarding "false and misleading" advertising practices. In 1965, the Federal Trade Commission launched additional hearings questioning the safety and efficacy of PPA-containing appetite suppressants. Though some evidence and clinical studies undermined PPA as an anorectic agent, the FTC examiner was not convinced by the research and recommended that PPA be considered an effective therapy. FDA advisory review panels reached similar conclusions in the late 1970s and early 1980s and, as a result, the FDA allowed the continued over-the-counter sale of PPA-containing products.[38] By the early 1980s, PPA was a key ingredient in more than seventy over-the-counter diet pill preparations and the fifth most used drug in the United States. At that point, Thompson was the market leader in diet aids, be they such appetite suppressants as Dexatrim and Appedrine or meal replacements like Slim-Fast, and its reaction to the backlash against its products was swift and sustained. Besides testimony before Congress defending diet pills, their efforts included an advertising blitz in the papers

---

* PPA ultimately became widely used as an orally administered nasal decongestant because it did not appreciably accelerate heart rate or elevate blood pressure and was substantially less stimulating to the central nervous system than ephedrine.

and on radio and television. By 1990, an estimated 16 billion PPA-containing products were consumed annually.[39] Generally, the diet drug industry was estimated to exceed $400 million and, according to certain estimates, 10 million Americans were regularly popping diet pills in the battle to become thin. Financial analysts, for their part, felt that diet products had plenty of room for market expansion.[40]

The FDA was also a crucial player in the debate over diet pills in the late 1970s and early 1980s. Prior to the election of Ronald Reagan and rampant discussion of a conservative revolution, the FDA's institutional identity was tested and toughened in the political and economic turmoil of the 1970s, as demonstrated in chapter 3.[41] Between 1974 and 1980, when the government first initiated studies and guidelines concerning weight loss and health, congressional scrutiny of the FDA reached prodigious heights. First, the agency was probed for what was perceived to be a damagingly close relationship with the pharmaceutical industry. Second, the drug lag, the label given for the unusually long time it required to approve a drug, brought the FDA a flood of criticism. Though the FDA rejected the term altogether, the "drug lag" sobriquet resonated and helped generate various congressional hearings as well as an enduring debate that carried over into the 1980s.[42] The Reagan administration's objective was to downsize the gatekeeper of the nation's drug supply, even though Reagan had offered surprisingly positive views of the agency's history and value to American society. He appointed moderate deregulators to manage the FDA and the Department of Health and Human Services (HHS) and fostered a healthy and accommodating relationship between the drug industry and the FDA. Moreover, in accordance with the example set by Jimmy Carter, Ronald Reagan continued to decrease FDA funds in fulfillment of his guarantee to reduce federal spending. Controlled for inflation, the FDA's budget remained static in the 1980s and the FDA suffered dwindling staff levels.[43]

The effort to trim down the size and authority of the FDA elicited a disapproving response from Congress and public interest groups.[44] According to Dr Sidney M. Wolfe, head of the Public Citizen Health Research Group and a man who would play a large role in the debate over diet pills, "We've seen a deterioration in the FDA's policing of the drug-medical device industry, and Americans are beginning to taste the fatal or health-destroying fruits of this partnership."[45] Representative John Dingell (D-MI) commented in December 1988, "This is a terrible mess, the denigration and emasculation of a fine and once-proud agency."[46] The FDA's chief, James S. Benson, also voiced his concern when he testified to a Department of Health and Human Services advisory committee. "We are *overdrawn* [italics mine] on virtually all accounts," Benson argued, and "FDA managers have been forced to cannibalize core functions and other programs to accommodate these new legislative activities."[47] Then, during the 1990s, there was an effort to rejuvenate the agency.*[48]

RISK ASSESSMENT

In the 1970s, even as obesity and weight loss garnered more attention as national issues, diet pills came under increasing scrutiny. Case reports emerged documenting hemorrhagic strokes in people – mainly women – who had taken various medications containing PPA. In 1979, an FDA advisory panel of doctors and scientists was assembled and established that PPA diet pills "may help people lose weight effectively." The panel also recommended that the FDA endorse a higher dosage.[49] This particular report failed to prove decisive, and officials at the agency "spent the next three years reviewing the panel's conclusions."[50]

This three-year delay was founded on various reasons: first, the absence of robust evidence supporting PPA; second, the strident argument against PPA coming from the medical community; and third, mounting anecdotal evidence in the medical literature underpinning the dangers of PPA.[51] Journalist Jane Brody has argued that the original 1979 decision was undermined by imperfect research. "The panel's opinion," she wrote, "was based on a number of unpublished, unnamed studies that the[se] advisers readily admitted were scientifically deficient."[52] Even worse, in 1981, Dr Albert Dietz, a clinical pharmacologist at the North Dakota School of Medicine, discovered that seven women were admitted to a hospital in Fargo, ND, suffering from anxiety, agitation, and dizziness. These patients of varying sizes and shapes were all taking diet pills containing PPA. While defending his review, published in the prominent *Journal of the American Medical Association* (JAMA), Dietz announced more research was immediately

---

* In particular, the Prescription Drug User Fee Act (PDUFA) was passed as part of the FDA Revitalization Act. It was an essential alteration of the status quo at the FDA, designed to inject the FDA with extra resources and accelerate the drug approval process.

required.[53] Alan Blum, president of Doctors Ought To Care, went a step further in April 1981 when he called for an outright ban on "the manufacture, sale and distribution" of products containing PPA. Six months after that, the Center for Science in the Public Interest (CSPI) and the National Women's Health Network (NWHN), consumer advocacy groups, publicly petitioned the FDA to disallow all dietary aids with PPA. Time, it seemed, was running short for PPA.

Yet, this was only the beginning of what would become a drawn-out and animated contest where individuals and institutions struggled mightily over the legitimacy of this pharmaceutical. In 1982, the FDA finally published the original 1979 advisory panel report and delayed a final decision on PPA, which "called for more research to determine a safe dose range."*[54] Following this decision, the issue of PPA's safety grew increasingly politicized in 1983 as Congress took up PPA's safety and efficacy. The House Select Committee on Aging, for example, focused almost exclusively on PPA during its 21 July hearing. Representative Mary Oakar (D-OH) declared that she had received several complaints from her constituents about adverse reactions; therefore, she decided that the FDA was neglectful "in not scrutinizing PPA." To authenticate her case about the dangers of PPA and the FDA's failure, Oakar convened a group of diet pill victims.

The hearings demonstrated no consensus of opinion. Reflecting the difficulty of the debate about PPA, another Democrat, Tom Lantos of California, raised a note of skepticism during the proceedings and about his colleague Oakar's approach. He stated his concern about the parade of victims, vilification of the drug industry, and lack of scientific evidence for the criticism of diet pills. He thought that to call out PPA was hazardous when such a claim was based on a "small number" of adverse reaction reports. In his view, this indicated sloppy reasoning and would prove to be a mistake. From his perspective, it was vital to consider "the many millions who benefit from these drugs" and adopt a balanced perspective on the risks and rewards. Lawmakers and regulators had to be cognizant of those who had benefited from diet pills as well as those harmed by them.[55]

Taking action on diet pills with PPA was not nearly as straightforward as banning starch blocker pills, where the evidence was clear

---

* In doing this, the FDA allowed PPA to be used at its current dosage level of 75 milligrams per day but ignored the panel's recommendation to double it to 150 milligrams.

and one-sided. During the July 1983 congressional hearings, for instance, the Center for Science in the Public Interest and Thompson Medical debated the available facts, which were anything but absolutely plain. While one witness asserted that "PPA was a fraud"[56] but added that gaps in research certainly existed, another witness testified that controlled studies of PPA's effect on blood pressure demonstrated mean elevations – even after a single dose.[57] At the same time, representatives of Thompson vigorously challenged the notion that PPA was unsafe and argued that the available evidence was scant. But this represented, in a microcosm, the company's attitude throughout the 1980s.[58]

In August 1983, a month after Mary Oakar's congressional hearing, Thompson was forced to pull nationwide advertisements for diet pills that the CSPI had called misleading. In the CSPI's view, the ads exaggerated weight-loss benefits and failed to disclose certain risks intrinsic to diet pills. For example, the fact that persons with high blood pressure or heart, thyroid, or kidney disease should not use pills containing PPA was omitted. Moreover, the ads erroneously claimed that Thompson products contained no stimulants. It appeared to be a non sequitur. And the courts agreed. The Ventura County District Attorney in California fined Thompson $145,000 for this false advertising.[59]

The company fought back. Thompson sought to publicly demonstrate the safety and efficacy of PPA in June 1984. The company sponsored a $100,000 two-day conference to investigate the available scientific evidence surrounding PPA, and a panel of twenty-one prominent scientists presented their mainly upbeat views on OTC diet pills. In certain instances, presenters rejected the notion that risk was involved with diet pills; in other cases, presenters argued against increased restrictions on PPA. According to Michael Weintraub, an expert in the field of clinical trials at the University of Rochester School of Medicine and Dentistry, "PPA has a modest, but consistent and definite effect in helping people to lose weight … the concurrence of evidence is quite positive."[60] Another expert, Donald Wesson, a drug specialist from Berkeley, agreed that the CSPI was wide of the mark in calling for more regulations. He stated that the effort to curb OTC diet aids was "misdirected."[61] Referring to the call for a ban on PPA, David Smith, from the University of California School of Medicine, proclaimed that such statements by the Center for Science in the Public Interest were "offensive."[62] John Morgan, the conference director, summed up the general finding of the meeting when he declared, "the reports of adverse reactions are largely unproven."[63]

On 11 June, the final day of the New York conference, the controversy and uncertainty over PPA aired on the Public Broadcasting Station's (PBS) *MacNeil/Lehrer NewsHour*. In a lively exchange, Bambi Young, of the CSPI, and Dr Harold Silverman, a member of the Massachusetts College of Pharmacy and a Thompson consultant, debated the safety, efficacy, and regulatory boundaries of PPA. When asked her outlook on diet pills containing PPA, Young tackled both their safety and effectiveness: "Our concerns," she began, "are that they are unsafe for a large fraction of the people who are likely to take them, that they don't really work for achieving significant weight loss, and that the way they're being advertised is seriously misleading."[64] The interviewer then asked Young to express the perils of diet pills. In Young's estimation, the medical community recognized that consumers should not take PPA products if they had high blood pressure, heart disease, thyroid disease, diabetes, or a number of other disorders. Yet, "interestingly enough," she argued, "most of the studies that have been offered in support of the safety of PPA diet pills were done on people who have been specifically excluded for those disorders." In her view, the scientific studies were not being conducted properly and it was not possible to accurately assess diet pills with PPA.

Silverman, who had participated in the two-day symposium, offered a stark alternative about the safety of PPA. From his perspective, Young was "overestimating a problem that really doesn't exist." The scientific evidence supported the safety of diet pills and, in addressing the protocols inherent in various studies, he obdurately held that he, not Young, was the scientific authority:

There are several thousand people who have now been very carefully studied. There are many, many people with medical problems who have now received the drug, [and] been very carefully studied. In other words, there is no threat to life or threat to death, as she indicates.[65]

An edgy exchange then unfolded, one that touched on the legitimacy and integrity of both participants' grasp of the scientific data. "It was my understanding," said Silverman, "that I knew all of the research that had been going on. And I'm quite familiar with the research that has been going on." Unwilling to let this go unanswered, Young claimed that her comprehension of the science was superior. "So am I. I just went to the FDA and looked at the record this afternoon and I checked the studies, and that's what they say."[66] Certainly, a lot was at stake.

As the interview neared completion, the effectiveness of PPA was disputed. Silverman proclaimed that "approximately a pound to a pound and a half of weight per week is lost when an individual takes this product," but Young argued that "an average consumer taking the diet aid can expect to lose roughly – well, less than half a pound a week if you correct for the placebo effect, which you need to do because the placebo effect is very powerful." Taking aim at Thompson's advertising techniques, Young continued, "I think the average consumer would not consider that effective if that information were clearly revealed."[67]

In the face of such critiques, Thompson continued to turn up the promotional heat and push back against such groups as the CSPI and Public Citizen. In 1985, Thompson named February "National Weight Loss" month. The company offered rebates, discounts, and bonus packs. According to *Business Week*, over $30 million was spent in this effort.[68] By the end of the year, revenues topped $137 million and Thompson possessed nearly 60 percent of the appetite suppressant and nutritional meal replacement markets.[69] Daniel Abraham, chairman of Thompson, stressed that Americans loved his products and proclaimed that Thompson received thousands of enthusiastic letters every year, many containing photographs illustrating weight loss. "The bottom line," stated Abraham in 1984, "is that people who use it like it."[70] Yet this promotional effort transcended mere consumer appreciation and engaged with fears of an interfering and meddlesome government. In a particularly one-sided article in *Consumer's Research* called "The Controversy over Diet Drugs," the attempt to study and perhaps place more regulations on PPA was exaggerated as "the cutting edge of a move to restrict all over-the-counter drugs."[71] The article also highlighted the greater risks of alcohol, aspirin, and acetaminophen compared to PPA. It then concluded by appealing to Americans' pocketbooks and concerns about an imperious and intrusive federal government. "Besides limiting consumers' choices, restrictions on relatively safe drugs will drive up costs."[72] If the legal boundaries of diet pills were altered – that is, if PPA was reclassified and made less acceptable – vulnerable and overweight American consumers would lose access to solutions they needed.

Dr John Morgan, a professor of pharmacology at City University of New York and the individual who had helped organize the New York conference, was especially instrumental in shaping views of diet pills with PPA. In 1985, he published a book called *Phenylpropanolamine: A Critical Analysis of Adverse Reactions and Overdosage*. The text reflected his skepticism of the theory that PPA elevated blood pressure and in this manner caused strokes. It was, in short, a book aimed at the critics of PPA. Of the swelling case reports and patient surveys, he wrote they resembled "metaphors" and were "unconvincing" as science.[73] He maintained that PPA met all of the criteria for over-the-counter medications and it was being unnecessarily demonized. Just as Dr Silverman had professed on national television, Morgan wrote that little risk was associated with these diet pills.[74]

Congress again addressed PPA in 1990, when Representative Ron Wyden (D-OR) convened hearings of the House Small Business Subcommittee on Regulation, Business Opportunities, and Energy. Dr Thaddeus Prout was front and centre. He also issued a challenge: "I defy anyone," he said, "to find another unregulated drug that has such a record of disaster." The FDA, he continued, was proving negligent by not moving more swiftly and convincingly against PPA.[75] The response from the agency was immediate. In 1991, the FDA's new commissioner, Dr David Kessler, responded to Prout's ultimatum and arranged for a public hearing on PPA. Held on 9 May, this event was designed to scrutinize the strokes in young women and first-time users.[76] To long-time followers of the PPA saga, the result of this FDA event mirrored the 1982 decision, when additional research was demanded; in short, a demonstrable association between PPA and hemorrhagic stroke would only be attained through "a large, carefully conducted study that might take years."[77] From the FDA's point of view, of course, this was the only procedure that could credibly resolve if PPA users were in actual fact at risk. The scientific and medical community, in short, needed to produce certainty with long-term research. Meanwhile, the FDA adopted the identical position it had in 1982: it would not remove diet pills from the OTC market until it had seen such research.[78]

By 1992, the major manufacturers of diet pills, Thompson Medical and Ciba-Geigy (later Novartis), initiated an extensive epidemiological study and enlisted two Yale University researchers, Dr Lawrence

Brass (a stroke expert) and Dr Ralph Horwitz (an epidemiologist), to design and carry out such an investigation. To outsiders, it appeared that the Yale Hemorrhagic Stroke Project (HSP) was going to be a rubber stamp. Thompson and Ciba-Geigy, as well as the Non-prescription Drug Manufacturers Association (later the Consumer Health Care Products Association), influenced certain "methodological decisions" when crafting the research plan. Similarly, researchers suspicious of the relationship between strokes and PPA were selected; and industry picked a chairman for the study's three-member oversight committee, Dr Louis Lasagna of Tufts University, who was on friendly terms with the diet pill manufacturers.[79] Brass, for his part, was initially very dubious of the connection between PPA and strokes. "My bias at the time," he stated, "was that the data for an association" was "weak."[80]

Years later, though, the Yale Stroke Project proved to be anything but rigged by the pharmaceutical industry. The investigation lasted from December 1994 until July 1999 and involved men and women recruited from 44 hospitals in 4 geographic regions of the United States.[81] The examination of 702 stroke cases in people 18 to 49 years old identified 27 victims, mostly women, who had taken PPA before their attack, and this was compared to a control group of 1,376 people. For all subjects, irrespective of gender, the risk of stroke increased by 50 percent, though this finding fell short of statistical significance.[82] The most disturbing finding was that women who had taken an appetite suppressant were 16 times more likely to have a stroke in three days than those in a control group who had not taken one.[83] Dr Brass, who had been previously skeptical, expressed astonishment at the link, while Dr Lasagna, who had once written so boldly about PPA's safety, approved the findings as head of the three-person oversight committee and instructed the researchers to contact the FDA without delay.[84] PPA truly was dangerous.

DECISION TIME

In October 1999, the FDA was presented with the Yale study's findings and an open meeting of its Nonprescription Drugs Advisory Committee (NDAC) was hastily scheduled.[85] On the surface, the HSP findings appeared solid and conclusive. Yet, even before the hearings took place, the diet pill industry players who had sponsored and developed the study sought to create uncertainty about its findings.[86]

The Consumer Health Care Products Association raised concerns about the design of the study that its group had contributed to years before. It also wanted to underscore PPA's overall safety record. Whereas the Center for Science in the Public Interest, as well as other groups, had promoted the uncertain safety of PPA, now the 119-year-old Consumer Health Care Products Association (CHPA) advocated in support of PPA by promoting the illegitimacy of the Yale study.

During the October meeting, medical experts from the industry-funded CHPA sought to cast doubt on the HSP and propose moderation on the part of the FDA. "I urge more research," declared one industry expert, rather than "any recommendation for a policy statement that is premature and unwarranted on the current totality of the evidence."[87] Another member of the CHPA review team said that the HSP produced additional uncertainty since "there are enough issues left open that it's very hard to make a judgment."[88] A third member brashly stated that the HSP was a "failed study."[89] Dr Sollers, who led the CHPA team, agreed and criticized the flimsy research findings. "The HSP Study does not provide the quality and the extent of scientific documentation necessary to support a change in [the] OTC status of PPA," he maintained, "because of inherent limitations, its small numbers of exposed cases and controls, inherent bias, inadequate control for confounding, [and] concerns about chosen statistical methods."[90] Sollers then highlighted the need for more research and suggested alternative, market-oriented pathways for the FDA. He declared that the FDA ought to ramp up surveillance measures through a policy of voluntary submission of adverse reactions from companies. "Companies," he asserted, "would be interested in working with [the] FDA to identify a procedure to do that."[91] Further, he argued that instead of exerting unwarranted control over the drug industry, the FDA should "finalize its labeling requirements" that call for information about maximum dosage and side effects.[92] He implied this would empower the consumer.

Following the argument made against the Yale Study, Dr Lois La Grande of the Food and Drug Administration mapped the history of PPA and responded to the skeptical CHPA group. During testimony that rebutted much of the critique, La Grande referred to the fact that the study had been "sponsored" by the CHPA and "the protocol was extensively reviewed on many occasions by Yale, the CHPA, and the agency."[93] Near the conclusion of Dr La Grande's report, she asserted that a "causal association" had been established by the study through

a "temporal relationship" and focus on "dose response."[94] What was
absent, unfortunately, was a second study to verify the findings. "The
question that we must ask ourselves," she ended, "is it in the public's
health interest to wait another 10 to 15 years so that this [study] could
be replicated or do we have so many other criteria fulfilled for causal
association?" Was there that much uncertainty?[95]

Dr Sidney Wolfe, the head of Public Citizen's Health Research
Group, one of the nation's more formidable health activism organizations, was also provided the opportunity to speak. Clearly frustrated, he underlined that the HSP study was not even necessary,
since "the literature back 10 years or more was clear enough." Wolfe
then ably summed up some of the absurdities of the contest over
PPA. He noted, for instance, that the same consultants employed by
the CHPA "before it signed off on the design and details of the study"
were now advancing the "methodologic criticisms" of the HSP. When
he shifted to the scientific approach, he added, "for every case control study, there are always those who find something wrong with
it because it lacks the perfection of randomized control trials."[96]
This meant there was an "extraordinarily skewed representation of
industry-funded critics there to say nay or maybe not."[97] Wolfe then
described what he viewed as the awesome power of the drug industry, of Big Pharma, to manipulate scientific knowledge:

> PPA is just another example in a long history of many serious
> public health hazards caused by drugs or medical devices which
> were allowed to continue endangering people much longer than
> they should after sufficient evidence for action was available
> because of industry-funded nit-picking with the methodology
> of the studies, often case control studies such as the one being
> discussed today.[98]

It was a nail in the coffin. After this final debate about the validity
of the science, the FDA drug panel finally sided with the researchers
and Yale's HSP. The panel's members determined that the study was
"well-designed" and "the investigators took reasonable steps to minimize bias and confounding." To eradicate any remaining doubts, the
FDA also declared, "the study had clear objectives and sound epidemiology practices were used in its design and execution."[99]

The final decision held, in short, that the benefits of the intended
uses of phenylpropanolamine did not outweigh the potential risk,

and PPA "was not considered to be generally recognized as safe."[100] More particularly, when asked whether phenylpropanolomine could be generally recognized as safe for use as an appetite suppressant, thirteen of the fourteen NDAC members voted that it could not. Additionally, twelve of the fourteen members agreed that PPA was not safe as a nasal decongestant either. Subsequently, the FDA leadership accepted the advice of the panel.[101] Afterward, one spokesperson from the FDA plainly discussed the strokes: "these are strokes in people who just should not be having them."[102] A 3 November 2000 letter signed by Janet Woodcock, the director of the Center for Drug Evaluation and Research, recommended that over a hundred products be removed from the market on a voluntary basis.[103] The drug was relegated to a different level of safety and efficacy – in essence, of legitimacy. Its career pathway changed, its regulatory status adjusted.

THE ROAD TO SLENDERNESS

Drug companies obeyed the FDA's order, but the issue continued to generate debate. According to an FDA official, industry hurt itself in the run-up to the hearings when "they essentially trashed the [HSP] study, even though they are the ones who designed it and financed it."[104] James Cope, a former president of the CHPA, told one reporter very bluntly, "We came out and said we don't like our own study. It's predictable: if the results don't come out the way you like ... you point out the weaknesses in it."[105] After the FDA's verdict, for example, a lawyer for Bayer Pharmaceuticals, Jerry Tottenham, argued, "We did not believe then, nor do we believe now, that PPA was dangerous." Tottenham reiterated doubts about the robustness of the evidence when he added that there was "no valid scientific evidence" of a link between strokes and PPA.[106] At the time of this statement, over 2,000 lawsuits were ongoing in the United States.

For over a century, vulnerable, gullible, and unsuspecting American consumers like Gloria Davis and Tricia Newenham have explored multiple medicines and techniques to combat overweight and obesity. In the 1970s, the House and Senate began to issue nutrition reports and dietary guidelines as health care costs associated with obesity steadily increased; nevertheless, the average American's reliance on and appetite for medical products that aided weight loss did not diminish.

Diet pills containing phenylpropanolamine acted as one of the more popular choices in the 1970s, 1980s, and 1990s. The debate over their safety and efficacy pitted multiple participants in the complex system of health product regulation against each other. Scientific consensus was up in the air, much as it was in the cases of LSD and Laetrile, and with cannabis now. Risks and rewards were hotly debated. In the case of Laetrile, which was a contemporaneous struggle over legitimacy and safety, the FDA required solid evidence – in short, a degree of certainty – as a basis for a final ruling, and all parties tried to influence the contest in congressional hearings, scholarly publications, newsprint, and on television. For all its support, though, Laetrile was a *single* product and did not have the weight of an entire self-help and dieting industry behind it. It possessed outsider status, and sought to move from the realm of illegitimacy to legitimacy. In a period that spanned over twenty years, various organizations and actors levelled charges and counter-charges advocating on behalf of weight-loss pills. This was to prevent a shift from the realm of acceptance to greater controls. For its part, the diet industry, on which Americans spent nearly $10 billion per year in the 1980s, was a significant force in the contest over the safety and effectiveness of pills.[107] When the five-year HSP study finally concluded, this, too, became the subject of significant interpretation, further illustrating the murkiness of scientific knowledge development in the midst of a climate of contrary pressures. The subject of PPA justifiably puzzled average Americans not always familiar with the particular jargon of scientific analysis or the differences between a case control study and a randomized controlled study, if they were even aware of it all.

"For many large Americans," according to journalist N.R. Kleinfield, "the road to slenderness was paved with diet pills."[108] In the 1990s, for example, Americans continued to take Fen-Phen, Pondimin, Redux, and other easily available diet drugs that were proven to be rather dangerous. Despite this, "neither scandals nor deaths nor fears of being duped dampen the consumer mania for thinness without pain."[109] Such debates have not abated. In February 2012, FDA officials began reviewing, for the second time, the safety of diet pill Qnexa, which has been linked to birth defects and heart problems.[110] *Consumer Reports* personnel point out that there are "an estimated 65,000 supplements on the markets" and "dietary supplement makers are not even required to register their products." It is a chilling thought that "[t]he FDA's only method of tackling the problem of adulterated supplements is to purchase them off the store shelves and test them one product at a time for drugs." Under the current regulatory regime, "[t]he FDA is playing a game of whack-a-mole with unscrupulous supplement makers, and it's putting consumers at risk." Worse still, weight-loss supplements aimed at the overweight continue to crop up containing dangerous drugs such as oxilofrine, a close relative of ephedrine.[111] There are nearly 1 billion overweight adults across the globe, with the US having the largest overweight and obese population. The most common method of fighting fat among this cohort has been "to use unhealthy weight management strategies (i.e., diet pills and laxatives) as opposed to engaging in healthier strategies." American dieters spent roughly $61 billion on such products in 2010 alone. Many of the products they bought contained toxic substances, including phenylpropanolamine (PPA). And "[w]ith the internet making even banned products readily accessible" it is nearly impossible to protect consumers.[112] As modern society continues to struggle with obesity, the history of diet pill regulation may continue to display familiar patterns. If this is the case, we ought to consider such pills alongside other strange medicines.

8

A KETAMINE CONCLUSION

Special K is not just a breakfast cereal and party drug. Also known as ketamine, it has long been used as an anesthetic in short-term diagnostic and surgical procedures.[1] But Special K is now driving a significant debate in mental health circles because a growing number of psychiatrists in the United States and elsewhere have been using it to combat depression. According to Andrew Pollack in the *New York Times*, "it is either the most exciting new treatment in years" or it's a "hallucinogenic drug that is wrongly being dispensed to desperate patients."[2] There is, as in all of the cases presented in this book, a decided lack of data necessary for any rational, evidence-informed decision. At this stage, the jury isn't even out. Yet, leading medical centres, including the National Institute of Health, Yale, and Oxford, are proposing that low-dose ketamine for major depression has tremendous potential. It has become, according to *Scientific American*, a rising star in the world of depression research.[3]

Ketamine works for roughly 75 percent of patients who have been unaffected by other forms of treatment, such as Prozac (which works in 58 percent of patients). Moreover, the time horizons involved with ketamine are glorified; it works in hours, sometimes even minutes, and its effects last for several weeks. According to *The Economist*, a single dose can reduce thoughts of suicide. As a consequence, while it has not formally been approved for use in treating depression, it is commonly prescribed "off label," and clinics have sprung up all over the United States, in particular, to offer infusions of the drug (which must be taken intravenously, if it is to work). Anecdotal reports have suggested that it has already saved many lives.[4]

Patrick Cameron, from Toronto, would agree. In 2013–14, he travelled to New York City on various occasions to visit private clinics for doses of ketamine, all in an effort to relieve his suffering from intractable depression. "This is the only thing that's worked," he noted. "I might have finally found the answer."[5] He had tried anti-depressant drugs and found them unhelpful. Ketamine was different. Still, the question of ketamine's efficacy remains controversial. As a result, it constitutes not only another drug in a long line of contested medicines for depression, but a further example of the struggle that either real or perceived recreational drugs face in navigating the blurry line of stigmatization and legitimacy.

Originally synthesized in the 1960s, ketamine acted as an alternative to phencyclidine (PCP or "angel dust") and users often found it produced altered physical, spatial, and temporal states. It grew as a recreational drug and, along with MDMA (Ecstasy), was bound up in rave culture. By 2006, the National Institute of Mental Health initiated the first controlled study of ketamine for treating depression. A virtual tidal wave of studies followed, many of which were promising. In the UK, the lead researcher of an Oxford-based study of twenty-eight people was effusive. "It really is dramatic for some people," said Dr Rupert McShane; "it's the sort of thing that really makes it worth doing psychiatry."[6] At the same time, the pharmaceutical industry has demonstrated interest in bringing ketamine products to the medical marketplace. AstraZeneca tried and then ceased developing a drug, whereas Johnson & Johnson is in the midst of trials for a nasal spray containing esketamine, a ketamine derivative. Allergan has also embarked on phase III trials on a ketamine-like antidepressant that it says has a rapid effect on major depressive disorder. There are other companies, including Baltimore's Cerecor, currently seeking to cash in on ketamine. For Kate Lyons in *The Guardian*, "once upon a time, the future of mental health treatment was drugs. The advent of Prozac and [a] whole class of similar medication in the 1990s gave doctors an easy option and big pharma easy money." Yet, twenty years on, the problems have not gone away. "In fact," she writes, "mental illness is much more pervasive, with depression now the world's second biggest cause of disability." With pharmaceutical pipelines rather dry, patients, physicians, and researchers – as well as drug company executives – are searching for prospects.[7] According to psychiatrist Ben Sessa, doctors, whether they are oncologists or psychiatrists, will "try any drug under the sun, any treatment ... they are scientists and they are humane people."[8]

Part of the push behind ketamine rested with failures in the pharmaceutical industry, various researchers explained. While new antidepressants proved very beneficial, they were largely "me too" drugs in that they exerted influence – by levels of monamines – over weeks, even as patients continued to suffer. In essence, they were retooled monoamine oxidase inhibitors and tricyclic antidepressants. It was thought ketamine might have a shorter lag time, which could improve overall public health. Though various caveats were offered on paper, the findings were certainly intriguing. "We found," the researchers noted, "a robust, rapid (hours), and relatively sustained (1 week) response to a single dose of the NMDA antagonist ketamine. Improvement in mood ratings for the course of the week was greater with ketamine than placebo." Conducted under the aegis of the National Institutes of Mental Health, the study's authors added: "to our knowledge, there has never been a report of any other drug or somatic treatment (ie, sleep deprivation, thyrotropin releasing hormone, antidepressant, dexamethasone, or electroconvulsive therapy) that results in such a dramatic rapid and prolonged response with a single administration." In short, these were significant outcomes.[9]

By 2014, studies from all over the world were exploring not just ketamine's efficacy in treating depression, as well as drug addictions, but also its proper mode of administration. In Australia, researchers supported "prior observations of rapid acute antidepressant effects of i.v. ketamine in individuals with treatment-resistant depression," although the IV method did not prove to have longer-lasting effects. This contrasted with previously published findings. On the other hand, ketamine has been tested as therapy for heroin addiction. A 2007 Russian study, for instance, built on similar research carried out in the 1950s and 1960s, which held that psychedelic-assisted psychotherapy might be an efficient treatment for alcoholism and addictions.[10] The effects of psychedelic psychotherapy, according to the researchers, are often very pronounced within several days or weeks after a treatment session, but then these effects quickly decline. This phenomenon was termed a "psychedelic afterglow." Accordingly, a trial was designed to examine the "profound transformative experiences" which often accompany ketamine doses. Results established that upon a one-year follow-up, survival analysis demonstrated a significantly higher rate of abstinence in the multiple

KPT group. That is, multiple doses, along with psychotherapy, proved more effective in treating heroin addiction.[11]

Yet, psychiatrists in the US are waiting for neither the scientific community nor the pharmaceutical industry to act. Some have already begun to establish clinics. With the ability to use ketamine off-label, some American doctors are charging patients like Patrick Cameron $3,000 for six IV infusions of the drug. With ketamine not yet available in Canada, Cameron, who has opted not to undergo electroconvulsive therapy (ECT), is stuck for options. Canada may have adopted a universal healthcare model, become a pioneer in medical marijuana, and chosen to legalize heroin on a limited basis, as we have seen in this book. However, Canadian physicians – without a licence from Health Canada – are restricted from offering ketamine as an alternative. When Zoloft or Lexapro fail and Canadian citizens choose to skip the electroshock route, they are forced elsewhere and become medical tourists. Much like Steve McQueen in the early 1980s or HIV/AIDS activists such as Ron Woodroof in *Dallas Buyers Club*, these Canadians have hard, very personal, and sometimes expensive choices to make as health consumers in the medical marketplace. Just like Mark Hauk in Saskatoon or Dr Gifford-Jones, who both promoted alternative medicines in their own ways, Canadians are occasionally turning away from approved drugs.

As in the case of LSD's revival in mental health or the use of heroin and Laetrile as legitimate medicines, there has been resistance to psychiatrists administering ketamine. For Stanford's Alan F. Schatzberg, it is crucial to be wise about ketamine. "Until we know more," he cautioned in the *American Journal of Psychiatry*, "clinicians should be wary about embarking on a slippery ketamine slope."[12] In 2017, the *AJP* once more chronicled the highs and lows of this emerging therapy. It raised issues about some clinics that employed questionable practices, including advertising booster infusions of ketamine for those patients who'd already had ten shots. Worse still, one clinic in Florida allowed patients to self-administer intranasally. "Since 2016, things have picked up," said psychiatrist Steve Levine, and "it scares the hell out of me that this is still unregulated."[13] Other warnings about ketamine are as follows. First, severely depressed patients have trouble weighing the risks and rewards associated with experimental therapies. Second, many clinics are run by anesthesiologists, who offer limited psychiatric treatment. Third, the rise of ketamine has detracted from the well-understood electroconvulsive therapy (ECT), which has, in many psychiatrists' view, a proven track record of success. Fourth, the majority of ketamine infusions are not covered by insurance, meaning vulnerable patients pay out of pocket ($400–1,000) for a generic product that has been available for almost fifty years. Fifth, and finally, ketamine infusion has been marketed to physicians as a means to create a quick income stream. These criticisms, of course, have their merits and faults. But in a larger sense, the discussion about ketamine illustrates how the public, the scientific community, and regulatory bodies in North America and beyond continue to struggle in negotiating the line separating licit and illicit drugs.

Ketamine is both unique and similar to other strange medicines, including medical marijuana, LSD, or heroin. Special K does not come with all the cultural and political baggage of these other drugs, and, as an anesthetic, has been a valuable tool within mainstream medicine. Yet, "an emerging body of evidence supports oral ketamine as an effective analgesic in cancer and chronic non-malignant pain." Likewise, "prescribers must remain vigilant," but "this should not deter appropriate prescribing any more than concern about heroin abuse should deter the use of morphine."[14] The World Health Organization (WHO) has recommended against the scheduling and excessive regulation of ketamine on several occasions – 2006, 2012, 2014, and 2015 – because, when used properly, the risk remains minimal. As one WHO official put it: "The medical benefits of ketamine far outweigh potential harm from recreational use." Moves to criminalize ketamine "could limit access to the only anaesthetic and pain killer available in large areas of the developing world." WHO director for essential medicines and health products Kees De Joncheere also drew an analogy between ketamine and morphine to explain his organization's position. "Placing substances under international control can often limit access to them for medical purpose," he argued. "Morphine was a case in point: even though it is inexpensive and one of the best substances available for pain management, in most countries availability and use are limited due to excessive regulation."[15] The WHO has included ketamine in its list of "essential medicines – substances that should be available to patients in any health system."[16] Researchers are not simply concerned with ketamine's use as an analgesic: "Ketamine is undergoing resurgence of interest for its potential uses ... in psychiatry for severe depression ... Restrictions on ketamine will limit the investigation of these potential treatment options."[17]

Here the medical community and scientific establishment are pitted against national governments and anti-drug lobbyists to ensure a few bad experiences with ketamine do not thwart attempts to develop new therapies.*[18] As *Scientific American* wrote in 2014, "new thinking is desperately needed to aid the estimated 14 million American adults who suffer from severe mental illness." The approach to ketamine in the United States and Canada may be a useful position from which to start developing that fresh thought.[19] Yet national governments are not wholly attentive to the public health and medical establishments. Advisors to David Cameron's Conservative–Liberal Democrat coalition (2010–15) recommended that, instead of easing restrictions on ketamine, they should be tightened, citing widespread abuse by the public, high levels of toxicity, and evidence of "acute psychological effects that include severe dissociation."[20] Illicit consumption of a drug with potential therapeutic value – both real and perceived – once again clearly influenced the regulation debate.

FINAL THOUGHTS

When Donald Rumsfeld, the US secretary of defense (2001–06), was asked whether reports that "no evidence of a direct link" between the Iraqi regime and terrorist organizations were true, he responded with a now famous phrase. He explained the difficulty inherent to decision-making based on imperfect information:

> Reports that say that something hasn't happened are always interesting to me, because as we know, there are known knowns; there are things we know we know. We also know there are known unknowns; that is to say we know there are some things we do not know. But there are also unknown unknowns – the ones we don't know we don't know. And ... it is the latter category that tend to be the difficult ones.[21]

Though maddeningly elliptical, the idea has merit. Foreign policy seems to hold lessons for medical science, albeit with a slightly

* For example, China continues to pressure the US "to place ketamine, an anesthetic widely abused in China, on a U.N.-maintained list of international controlled substances."

different emphasis. The histories of the drugs recounted in this book demonstrate that the "unknown unknowns" do not dissuade the sick, dying, or curious from experimenting with drugs. Meanwhile, the cautious set warn of the "known unknowns," apprehensive that unverified, unsanctioned treatments will produce more harm than good. Yet, the "known knowns" are most salient in medicine, as pain and suffering are felt immediately, pushing desperate patients, advocates, and researchers to implore for compassion and institutional support in the fight for their relief.

The politics and policies of heroin in end-of-life settings between two neighbours, Canada and the United States, illustrate this. In the 1980s, Americans wrangled over the efficacy of heroin but legislators also employed fearful language about heroin infiltrating the streets. Meanwhile, heroin for the dying was made available further north in Canada, arguably because the influence of the UK provided the medical legitimacy – that perhaps heroin was not so strange after all. A recently elected Conservative government thus chose an alternative path from conservative Republican policy-makers in the US. Laetrile as a cancer drug was equally contested, stimulating activists and medical entrepreneurs into action. It offered hope of a cure whereas heroin offered respite from pain. This was a crucial difference. Not only that, Laetrile's support was often based on broader claims about freedom in the medical marketplace. The science was muddy, but to hardcore advocates this didn't entirely matter. Choice and individualism were the core principles. Authority, in other words, ought to rest with the consumer-patient.

As we have seen, the struggle over the strangeness of medicines often pitted mainstream medical practitioners against interlopers, such as botanical healers, homeopaths, or medical cannabis dispensaries. Quackery has been around since the beginning of professional medicine. Legitimate and upstanding physicians did not want their field tainted by eccentrics without formal medical training. Yet, many debates have been intra-professional, characterized by acrimonious infighting and struggles within the field. It has not always been a struggle against barbarians at the gate. Just think about Dr Oz being criticized by his colleagues for advocating the use of unproven diet remedies. Or how legislators and regulators laboured over decisions about dangerous diet pills. Or LSD dividing basic researchers and clinicians. Or more current discussions about the wholesale use of cannabis in universal medical practice.

More broadly, the history of strange medicine is not simply about the perception and authorization of alternative products in the marketplace, nor just about the difficulties faced by marginal groups – the rebels on the fringes. As the preceding chapters have shown, it's about collective action, empowerment, and individualism, as well as expertise and evidence-based practices. It's complicated further by political ideologies and national interest, diagnostic difficulties and contested science. All of these factors influence how a well-accepted medicine might move into a peripheral outsider category or vice versa. A single product (such as cannabis) is different from a set of products (Canadian pharmaceuticals), of course, yet it's valuable to initiate the discussion. Drug products, in short, occupy interstitial spaces and may be remodelled as political, economic, and social circumstances require.

The historian Joseph M. Gabriel has elucidated how drug regulation came to incorporate not just the legal trade in pharmaceuticals but the black market in contraband, too. From the nineteenth century on, American lawmakers have tried to balance product safety with free markets in the interests of the consumer, who was willing to do just about anything to relieve their pain and suffering. Gabriel's argument has focused on pharmaceutical products and he has argued that this "complex dialectic" is "one in which individual freedom and social prohibition enacted through regulation are intertwined and mutually constitutive."[22] Accordingly, the exercise of choice in the consumption of medicine and medical services has often conflicted with the beliefs, methods, and authority of physicians, scientists, and regulators. The push and pull of this process, the control and resistance, gave birth to the modern medical marketplace and its regulation – and it is apparent in the illicit substances and contested pharmaceuticals discussed in this book.

This book has also embodied the different kinds of economic strategies and health systems in medicine. Patients have been portrayed as tourists and active decision-makers who have sought out alternative products and medicines in the marketplace. The chapters of this book have played with these themes, meanwhile positioning previously solitary drugs into conversation with each other. The rise of the empowered patient-consumer, who purportedly knows what is best for him- or herself and regards the physician in an instrumental manner, forms a vital part of *Strange Trips*. Supporters of the patient-consumer include advocacy groups, pharmaceutical companies, and free-market fundamentalists. Sometimes they are senior citizens travelling – as medical tourists – to Canada for a bargain. Other times they are unsatisfied with standard, approved painkillers and search for alternatives such as cannabis in dispensaries. Or, as in the case of diamorphine, they advocate for access to whatever opioid painkiller they wish. The patient-consumer might travel to Mexico, as Steve McQueen did. On occasion, too, respectable drugs shift into less reputable territory, when the border patrol, federal regulators, and non-governmental organizations debate the safety and efficacy of approved pills. Such patients have argued that excessive red tape causes "drug lag," thereby harming patients and imposing "unnecessary costs on a vibrant industry" and consumers. They have connected this – both correctly and incorrectly – to the "individual patient and his or her experience with disease and therapy" when mobilizing activists to push for increased access to new remedies. Regulators have responded by stressing the risks an overly liberal regime poses to public health and consumer protection.

Still, the concepts of freedom and choice have come to govern the discussion, and those who control the "symbolic language" of the debate have often carried the day on drug policy. Many of the groups that have successfully pressured government to ease restrictions on developing drugs have done so whether or not the medical establishment or scientific research supports the use of a given medicine.[23] What are doctors and regulators to do when they are under intense public scrutiny and patients are begging for relief? One British commentator described physicians "as helpless in the face of a population of patients who have an overwhelming need to alter chemically their experiences of the world in which they live." He compared the GP "to a barmaid in a gin shop … not only do patients know exactly what they want but … they usually get it."[24] Thomas Szasz, the controversial psychiatrist, believed this was as it should be. He called for patients to reject "the claim that the state has legitimate authority to tell us what substances we can or cannot ingest, or can make ingesting substances contingent on obtaining prior permission from agents of the state (that is, a doctors 'prescription')."[25] The right to autonomy and liberty, for him, superseded the nanny-state's overbearing designs. As governments in the United States and Canada faced an opioid crisis in 2015–17, one must question the value of such claims.

Besides just questions, though, it is also worth advancing a few final thoughts and recommendations. The first is to recognize how

drugs "have been central to the formation of civilizations, the definition of cultural identities, and the growth of the world economy."[26]
Of course, humans have been using psychoactive substances for
thousands of years. Evidence from across the pre-modern world
indicates the consumption of a variety of substances including wine,
tea leaves, peyote, cinchona bark, and various others, for a host of
medicinal, religious, and recreational purposes. A second thought
has to do with how we regard science in society. In particular, the
best way to treat science is as a fluid, intermediated (often very political) process. The different chapters of this book have demonstrated
this process. Such a view does not mean I have less faith in science,
but we ought to be aware of its potential fallibilities, in addition to
its strengths. Lastly, scholars, policy-makers, and politicians need to
be far less arrogant about the creation of policy. This will require
wider acknowledgment that rules and regulations are empirically
based, but also that they are a mirror image of cultural beliefs, political environments, economic realities, innovative technologies, and
further factors. Chapters in this book have shown, for instance, how
international, national, and local policies can diverge across time
and space. Even when they are analogous, policies may be *enforced*
differently. Relationships between humans and drugs – between regulators and the public – are overwhelmingly dependent on context.
Societies may evolve or regress, and so do attitudes, (mis)uses, and
understandings of drugs.

There are other concrete recommendations to make. The first section of this book focused on end-of-life therapies. Since the 1980s,
"considerable advances have been made" in the knowledge of the
management of symptoms in terminal illnesses – improvements that
warrant widespread incorporation into the clinical practice of both
generalists and specialists. The information about "comfort care" in
treating various symptoms and dealing with pain in terminal patients
is of the utmost importance.[27] As part of this, we ought to think more
about pain – that is, tackling the root causes of pain – instead of simply focusing on painkillers and addiction to these drugs. This might
be problematic amid an opioid crisis, but recalibrating public and
private discussions would be worthwhile. Relatedly, the treatment
of pain, among other factors, has led to a rise in medical tourism.
Decision-making around outbound medical travel typically involves
a range of information sources, and, whether one happens to be
dealing with antidepressant treatments, arthritis, or arthroscopy, the

internet plays a key role (as does information from informal networks of friends and peers). Studies suggest that medical tourists often pay more attention to soft information than hard clinical information, and there is little effective regulation of information.[28] As this book has shown, medical tourism is linked with patient empowerment, medical evidence, and the price of health services, such as access to ketamine. I recommend more studies of globalizing forces (transnational and national companies, World Health Organization guidelines, and in-country medical services) in conjunction with consumerism, advertising, and international drug regulation.

Lastly, public health officials often urge caution to drug-takers, and are frequently concerned that evidence buttresses the management of a given substance, either therapeutically or recreationally. They crave facts – more knowledge – before endorsing or outright rejecting any particular drug. In Aldous Huxley's dystopian novel *Brave New World* (1932), the hallucinogen soma controlled the population. Mustapha Mond, one of the regime's élites, explained the difficulty of coping with modern life and the necessity of altering the mind to avoid pain: "if ever, by some unlucky chance, anything unpleasant should happen, why, there's always *soma* to give you a holiday from the facts ... [and] to make you patient and long-suffering."[29] Similarly, the drugs described in this book have been heralded as providing relief from suffering – physical and psychic – and many have attested that they work. Yet, unlike soma, not one of them offers "a holiday from the facts," and it is the battle over the facts – not truths – that has set patients against doctors, lobbyists against public health officials, and pharmaceutical companies against regulators. Facts may not be understood the way they once were, making medicines very strange. In many cases, the science may be far from settled, but this has not prevented individuals from demanding access to and consuming untested and unconventional substances. Those involved in these debates will continue to push boundaries, resist change, and attempt to revolutionize medicine, rendering some drugs legitimate, others illegitimate, and many contested. The dialectic, and the strangeness, continues to unfold. I recommend getting used to this.

NOTES

INTRODUCTION

1 Chasin, *Assassin of Youth*, 6. See Pembleton, *Containing Addiction*.

2 Rotunda, "Savages to the Left of Me, Neurasthenics to the Right, Stuck in the Middle with You," 50–2.

3 Donald MacPherson, "Too Many Politicians Suffer from Drug Policy Abuse," *Huffington Post*, 11 November 2014, http://www.huffingtonpost.ca/donald-macpherson/drug-policy-conservatives_b_6136592.html. See also Small and Drucker, "Policy Makers Ignoring Science and Scientists Ignoring Policy," 16; Comeau et al., "News @ a Glance," 1336; Eggerston, "Health Minister Ends Special Access to Prescription Heroin," E773.

4 Geoff Mulgan, "Experts and Experimental Government," *The Guardian*, 5 April 2013, http://www.theguardian.com/science/political-science/2013/apr/05/experts-experimental-government.

5 A.I. Leshner, "The National Institute on Drug Abuse: Changes, Challenges, and Opportunities in 1996," in Harris, ed., *Problems of Drug Dependence 1996*, 12.

6 Nutt, *Drugs without the Hot Air*; Pallab Ghosh, "Mind-Altering Drugs Research Call from Prof David Nutt," *BBC News*, 23 January 2012, http://www.bbc.com/news/health-16678322; *David Nutt's Blog: Evidence, Not Exaggeration*, https://profdavidnutt.wordpress.com.

7 New scholarship that showcases how drugs influence science, culture, and war includes Kaiser and McCray, eds., *Groovy Science*, and Kamienski, *Shooting Up*.

8 Collins and Pinch, *Dr. Golem*.

9 Kuzmarov, "From Counter-Insurgency to Narco-Insurgency," 344–78.

10 See also Acker, *Creating the American Junkie*, and Schneider, *Smack*.

11 Nunn, "Race, Crime and the Pool of Surplus Criminality," 386–91;
    Loizeau, *Nancy Reagan: The Woman behind the Man*.

12 Loizeau, *Nancy Reagan in Perspective*, 105.

13 See especially Snelders et al., "On Cannabis, Chloral Hydrate, and
    Career Cycles of Psychotropic Drugs in Medicine," 95–114, and
    Musto, *The American Disease*.

14 Cayleff, *Nature's Path*, 275.

15 Pieters and Snelders, "From King Kong Pills to Mother's Little
    Helpers," 94.

16 See Nunn, "Race, Crime and the Pool of Surplus Criminality,"
    386–91.

17 David Farrar, "Chief Science Adviser Attacks Academic 'Arrogance'
    on Policy," *Times Higher Education*, 5 October 2017, 9.

18 Goode and Nachman, *Moral Panics*, 81; Cornwell and Linders, "The
    Myth of 'Moral Panic,'" 307–30; Horwitz, "Understanding
    Deregulation," 139–40.

19 For a discussion of consumer protection and regulations in the realm
    of the pharmaceutical industry, see Gabriel, *Medical Monopoly*;
    Greene, *Generic*; Li, *Blockbuster Drugs*.

20 Kuhn et al., *Buzzed*, 3.

21 "End the Ban on Psychoactive Drug Research," *Scientific American*,
    1 February 2014, http://www.scientificamerican.com/article/
    end-the-ban-on-psychoactive-drug-research/.

22 Sismondo, *America Walks into a Bar*; Malleck, *Try to Control
    Yourself*; McGirr, *The War on Alcohol*; Brandt, *The Cigarette
    Century*. See Rorabaugh's *Prohibition*.

23 Herzberg, "Entitled to Addiction?" 586–623; Greene and Herzberg,
    "Hidden in Plain Sight," 793–803.

24 Michaels, "Manufactured Uncertainty," 150. For more on risk, sci-
    ence, and decision-making, see Breyer's *Breaking the Vicious Circle*.

25 Li and Cui, "Patients without Borders," 20–1. See also Cohen et al.,
    eds., *Nudging Health*, and Hodges et al., eds., *Risks and Challenges
    in Medical Tourism*.

26 Stein, *Pivotal Decade*, viii–x; Richert, "Surveying the Seventies,"
    649–54.

27 "Legalising Pot in Canada: Justin Trudeau and the Cannabis
    Factory," *The Economist*, 19 December 2015, http://www.
    economist.com/news/

americas/21684186-converting-medical-marijuana-industry-recreational-one-will-not-be-easy-justin-trudeau.

28 Ben Spurr, "Legalizing Pot Will Be a Process of Trial and Error, U.S. Expert Warns Trudeau," *Toronto Star*, 25 October 2015, https://www.thestar.com/news/canada/2015/10/25/legalizing-pot-may-give-trudeau-headaches-us-expert.html.

29 John Ivison, "Canada Pot? How Mail-Order Marijuana Could Help Save the Struggling Post Office," *National Post*, 17 January 2016, http://news.nationalpost.com/full-comment/could-canada-post-become-canada-pot; Sylvain Charlebois, "For Canadian Pharmacies, Pot Is a Gateway Drug with High Upside," *Globe and Mail*, 24 February 2016, http://www.theglobeandmail.com/report-on-business/rob-commentary/for-canadian-pharmacies-pot-is-a-gate-way-drug-with-high-upside/article28866161/; Dan Malleck, "Why Should Liquor Control Boards Manage Weed Sales? They Already Know How," *Globe and Mail*, 15 December 2015, http://www.theglobeandmail.com/opinion/why-should-liquor-control-boards-manage-weed-sales-they-already-know-how/article27757191/; Lee Fang, "Alcohol Industry Bankrolls Fight Against Legal Pot in Battle of the Buzz," *The Intercept*, 15 September 2016, https://theintercept.com/2016/09/14/beer-pot-ballot/.

30 *The Lancet Psychiatry* 4, no. 5 (May 2017): 347–426.

CHAPTER ONE

1 Peter McKnight, "As B.C. Heroin Flap Shows, Drug Laws Are Not about Improving Health," *Globe and Mail*, 28 November 2014, http://www.theglobeandmail.com/globe-debate/as-bc-heroin-flap-shows-drug-laws-are-not-about-improving-our-health/article21824587/; Andrea Woo, "Vancouver Addicts Soon to Receive Prescription Heroin," *Globe and Mail*, 22 November 2014, http://www.theglobeandmail.com/news/british-columbia/vancouver-heroin-addicts-authorized-to-get-drug/article21717642/.

2 For a discussion of consumer protection in the realm of the pharmaceutical industry, see Richert, *Conservatism, Consumer Choice, and the Food and Drug Administration during the Reagan Era*.

3 Carnwath and White, *Heroin Century*, 148.

4 Bridget Kinsella, "Lessons from Canada Legalizing Heroin for Medicine," DPF: *Drug Policy Letter*, 22 April 1989, http://www.

drugtext.org/Drug-Policy-Letter-march/april-1989/lessons-from-canada-legalizing-heroin-for-medicine.html.

5 Joe Holley, "Judith Quattlebaum; Was an Advocate for Patients," *Washington Post*, 18 September 2004, http://www.washingtonpost.com/wp-dyn/articles/A30437-2004Sep17.html.

6 Walker, "How a Medical Journalist Helped to Legalize Heroin in Canada," 143.

7 Gifford-Jones, *You're Going to Do What?* 185.

8 Ibid., 182. See also Richert, "Heroin in the Hospice," E1231–2.

9 Gifford-Jones, *You're Going to Do What?* 174–5.

10 Ibid.

11 See Acker, *Creating the American Junkie*, and Schneider, *Smack*.

12 Lon Appleby, "The Big Fix," *Saturday Night*, November 1985, 15.

13 Da Sylva, "The CMA's Stand on the Medical Use of Heroin," 1515.

14 Appleby, "The Big Fix," 14.

15 Gifford-Jones, *You're Going to Do What?* 174.

16 Ibid.

17 Mattingly and Conley, "The Medical Prescription of Heroin for Terminal Cancer Patients," 337–54. See also Mold, *Heroin*.

18 Twycross, "Stumbling Blocks in the Study of Diamorphine," 309–13; Twycross, "Clinical Experience with Diamorphine in Advanced Malignant Disease," 184–98; Twycross, "Choice of Strong Analgesic in Terminal Cancer," 93–104.

19 Quoted in William F. Buckley Jr, "Mrs. Q: The Pain Killer," *National Review*, 11 July 1980, 861.

20 Duffin, "Palliative Care," 205–28.

21 Ibid., 210–11.

22 Claudia Wallis, Patricia Delaney, and Ruth Mehrtens Galvin, "Heroin, a Doctors' Dilemma," *Time* 123, no. 25 (11 June 1984): 62–3.

23 Kaplan, *The Hardest Drug*; Dale Beckett, "Heroin: The Gentle Drug," *New Society*, 26 July 1979, 181–2.

24 Clark, *To Comfort Always*.

25 Paradis and Cummings, "The Evolution of Hospice in America," 370–86.

26 Duffin, "Palliative Care," 211.

27 John Walsh, "The Enduring Mystery of Pain Measurement," *The Atlantic*, 10 January 2017, https://www.theatlantic.com/health/archive/2017/01/finding-a-language-for-pain/512615/.

28 Walker, "How a Medical Journalist Helped to Legalize Heroin in Canada," 144.

29 See Foley, "Controversies in Cancer Pain," 2259.

30 Gérald Lafrenière and Leah Spicer, *Illicit Drugs in Canada 1980–2001: A Review and Analysis of Enforcement Trends, Prepared for the Special Senate Committee on Illegal Drugs*, Library of Parliament, 26 June 2002, http://www.parl.gc.ca/Content/SEN/Committee/371/ille/library/DrugTrends-e.htm.

31 Gifford-Jones, *You're Going to Do What?* 191–3.

32 Walker, "How a Medical Journalist Helped to Legalize Heroin in Canada," 144.

33 Ibid.

34 "Heroin for Cancer: A Great Non-issue of Our Day," 1449–50.

35 Scott and Sellers, *Cancer Pain, A Monograph*.

36 Kinsella, "Lessons from Canada."

37 W. Gifford-Jones, "Foundation Seeks Support," *Globe and Mail*, 4 April 1983, 13.

38 Appleby, "The Big Fix," 16.

39 Ibid.

40 *Globe and Mail*, 17 December 1984, 9.

41 Appleby, "The Big Fix," 16.

42 Kinsella, "Lessons from Canada."

43 Appleby, "The Big Fix," 16.

44 Kinsella, "Lessons from Canada."

45 Scott and Sellers, *Cancer Pain*.

46 Appleby, "The Big Fix," 16.

47 Dorothy Lipovenko, "Panel Rejects Use of Heroin as Painkiller," *Globe and Mail*, 5 September 1984, M2.

48 Appleby, "The Big Fix," 17–18; Ghent, "Heroin," 811.

49 Legislative Assembly of Ontario, "Therapeutic Use of Heroin," Hansard Transcripts, Official Records for 18 October 1984, http://www.ontla.on.ca/web/house-proceedings/house_detail.do?locale=en&Parl=32&Sess=4&Date=1984-10-18#P419_131663.

50 Ibid.

51 Appleby, "The Big Fix," 13.

52 Ibid., 18.

53 Ibid.

54 Ibid.

55 Judith Quattlebaum, "Letters – Medical Establishment Blocks Pain Treatment," *New York Times*, 1 February 1980, A30.

56 James McCarthy, "The Doctor from Wales Who Slashed Crime and Drug Addiction – by Giving Out Heroin," *WalesOnline*, 20 June 2015, http://www.walesonline.co.uk/news/wales-news/doctor-heroin-slashed-crime-addiction-9495143; Hari, *Chasing the Scream*.

CHAPTER TWO

1 Burroughs, *Junkie*; Robert J. Dole Senate Papers–Legislative Relations, 1969–1996, Series 6, Box 130, Folder 3, Robert J. Dole Archive and Special Collections, University of Kansas, Lawrence, KS.
2 Holley, "Judith Quattlebaum."
3 Wailoo, *Pain*. See also Bourke, *The Story of Pain*; Thernstrom, *The Pain Chronicles*; Foreman, *A Nation in Pain*; Wall, *Pain*; Scarry, *The Body in Pain*.
4 See, for example, Boyd, *From Witches to Crack Moms*, 217–18; Courtwright, *Dark Paradise*, 62–82; Hickman, "Drugs and Race in American Culture," 71–91.
5 Nunn, "Race, Crime and the Pool of Surplus Criminality," 386.
6 Kaplan, *The Hardest Drug*; Beckett, "Heroin: The Gentle Drug."
7 Brecher, *Licit and Illicit Drugs*.
8 See Kuhn et al., *Buzzed*, 3.
9 Carnwath and White, *Heroin Century*, 148.
10 Schulman and Zelizer, eds., *Rightward Bound*; Farber and Bailey, eds., *America in the 1970s*; Jenkins, *Decade of Nightmares*; Kalman, *Right Star Rising*; Killen, *1973 Nervous Breakdown*; Schulman, *The Seventies*.
11 Gapstur and Thun, "Progress in the War on Cancer," 1084–5.
12 Drake, "Forty Years On," 757.
13 Richard Harris, "Why the War on Cancer Hasn't Been Won," *NPR*, 23 March 2015, http://www.npr.org/sections/health-shots/2015/03/23/394132747/why-the-war-on-cancer-hasnt-been-won.
14 Ibid.
15 Drake, "Forty Years On," 757. See also Siddhartha Mukherjee's *The Emperor of All Maladies: A Biography of Cancer* (London: Fourth Estate, 2011).
16 Holden, "Drug Abuse 1975," 638–41. See also Wilson, Moore, and Wheat, "The Problem of Heroin" and "Kids and Heroin: The Adolescent Epidemic," *Time* 95, no. 11 (16 March 1970): 20.
17 Kuzmarov, "From Counter-Insurgency to Narco-Insurgency."

18 Holden, "Drug Abuse 1975," 638–9.

19 James Q. Wilson, "The Fix," *The New Republic*, 25 October 1982, 24–9.

20 Richert, "'Therapy Means Political Change, Not Peanut Butter,'" 104–21.

21 Torrens, ed., *Hospice Program and Public Policy*, 8.

22 Paradis and Cummings, "The Evolution of Hospice in America."

23 Ibid.

24 Buckingham, "Hospice and Health Policy," 303–15.

25 Foster, "How Social Work Can Influence Hospital Management of Fatal Illness," 30–5. See also Daratsos and Howe, "The Development of Palliative Care Programs in the Veterans Administration: Zelda Foster's Legacy," 29–39.

26 Dennis Hasveni, "Zelda Foster, 71, Pioneer in Hospice Care," *New York Times*, 13 July 2006, B7.

27 Newman, "Elisabeth Kubler-Ross," 627.

28 Gill, "Hospice Pioneer," 18.

29 Paradis and Cummings, "The Evolution of Hospice in America."

30 Wailoo, *Pain*, 4.

31 Ibid.

32 Ibid.

33 Wallis et al., "Heroin, a Doctors' Dilemma," 62–3.

34 Kaplan, *The Hardest Drug*; Beckett, "Heroin: The Gentle Drug."

35 Wallis et al., "Heroin, a Doctors' Dilemma," 62.

36 Ibid.

37 Foreman, *A Nation in Pain*, 4.

38 Ibid.

39 Quoted in William F. Buckley Jr, "Mrs. Q: The Pain Killer," *National Review*, 11 July 1980, 861.

40 "Buckley Correspondence with Geri Cleary," 21 May 1985. Robert J. Dole Senate Papers–Legislative Relations, 1969–1996, Series 6, Box 676, Folder 2, Robert J. Dole Archive and Special Collections, University of Kansas, Lawrence, KS.

41 William F. Buckley Jr, "Drugs Drugs Everywhere – And No Solution in Sight," *National Review*, 9 August 1985, 54–5.

42 Ibid.

43 US Congress, House of Representatives, Committee on Interstate and Foreign Commerce, *Drug Regulation Reform – Oversight, New Drug Approval Process: Hearings Before the Subcommittee on*

Health and the Environment of the, House of Representatives, 96th Congress, 25 June 1980, 1–20.

44 Irvin Molotsky, "This Odd Couple Focuses on Health," *New York Times,* 14 September 1984, A24; Richert, *Conservatism, Consumer Choice, and the Food and Drug Administration,* 136–8. See also Hatch Memo, 29 October 1981, Legislative Files, Box 130, Folder 3, Robert J. Dole Archive.

45 Ibid.

46 "The Value in Heroin," *New York Times,* 23 July 1984, A18.

47 Hatch Memo, 29 October 1981, Legislative Files, Box 130, Folder 3, Robert J. Dole Archive.

48 Quattlebaum Letter, 9 Dec 1981, Legislative Files, Box 130, Folder 3, Robert J. Dole Archive.

49 Twycross, "Clinical Experience with Diamorphine."

50 Lewis and DiVita, "Is There a Place for Heroin in the Symptomatic Support of Cancer Patients?"; Boerner et al., "The Metabolism of Morphine and Heroin in Man," 63.

51 "Heroin and Cancer Pain," *Science News* 119, no. 20 (16 May 1981): 312.

52 Kaiko et al., "Analgesic and Mood Effects of Heroin and Morphine in Cancer Patients with Postoperative Pain," 1501–5.

53 Sun, "Heroin, Morphine Found Comparable as Pain-Killer," 277.

54 Wallis et al., "Heroin, a Doctors' Dilemma," 62–3.

55 Lasagna, "Heroin: A Medical Me-Too," 1539–40.

56 Sun, "Heroin, Morphine Found Comparable as Pain-Killer," 277.

57 Buckley Letter, 13 May 1982, Legislative Files, Box 130, Folder 3, Robert J. Dole Archive.

58 Blanchard Randall, "Heroin: Legalization for Medical Use," 24 July 1984, CRS-4, Library of Congress, Congressional Research Services, Science Policy Research Division, Washington, DC.

59 Arnold Trebach, "Relieve Pain with Heroin," *Washington Post,* 10 August 1984, A24.

60 Wallis et al., "Heroin, a Doctors' Dilemma," 62–3.

61 "Heroin for Cancer: A Great Non-issue of Our Day," *The Lancet,* 1449–50.

62 Wilson, "The Fix," 29.

63 Schneider, *Smack,* 170.

64 Kaplan, *The Hardest Drug,* 218.

65 Nunn, "Race, Crime and the Pool of Surplus Criminality," 390–2.

66 Wilson, "The Fix," 29.

67 Trebach, *The Great Drug War*, 292–3.
68 William F. Buckley Jr, "Pending Bill Legalize Heroin for the Sick," *Philadelphia Enquirer*, 29 September 1987, http://articles.philly.com/1987-09-29/news/26212037_1_heroin-cancer-patients-supply-of-illegal-drugs.
69 Arnold Trebach, "Relieve Pain with Heroin."
70 Trebach, *The Great Drug War*, 292.
71 Ibid.
72 Quoted in Stoll, "Why Not Heroin?" 173–94.
73 Trebach, *The Great Drug War*, 293. See also US Congress, House of Representatives, Subcommittee on Health and the Environment, *Compassionate Pain Relief Act: Hearings on H.R. 4762*, 98th Congress, 1985.
74 "Kids and Heroin: The Adolescent Epidemic," *Time* 95, no. 11 (16 March 1970): 20–8.
75 Trebach, *The Great Drug War*, 293.
76 Holley, "Judith Quattlebaum; Was an Advocate for Patients."
77 Quattlebaum, "Letters – Medical Establishment Blocks Pain Treatment."

CHAPTER THREE

1 Hawthorne, *Inside the* FDA, 51; Hilts, *Protecting America's Health*, 237; Richert, *Conservatism, Consumer Choice, and the Food and Drug Administration*.
2 Bill Minutaglio, "The Real Legacy of the Real Dallas Buyers Club Is That It Didn't Really Have One," *The Guardian*, 2 March 2014, http://www.theguardian.com/commentisfree/2014/mar/02/real-dallas-buyers-club-matthew-mcconaughey-character; Dylan Matthews, "What 'Dallas Buyers Club' Got Wrong about the AIDS Crisis," *Washington Post*, 10 December 2013, https://www.washingtonpost.com/news/wonk/wp/2013/12/10/what-dallas-buyers-club-got-wrong-about-the-aids-crisis/; Kyle Smith, "How the Oscar Winning Libertarian Favorite 'Dallas Buyers Club' Exposes the FDA," *Forbes*, 5 March 2014, http://www.forbes.com/sites/kylesmith/2014/03/05/how-the-oscar-winning-libertarian-favorite-dallas-buyers-club-exposes-the-fda/#18bc30629b5b.
3 Engel, *The Epidemic*; Shilts, *And the Band Played On*.
4 Mark Gevisser, "Battling the FDA: AIDS Movement Seizes Control," *The Nation* 247, no. 19 (19 December 1988): 677–9; Richard

Seltzer, "Protestors Hit FDA for AIDS Drug Policies," *Chemical and Engineering News* 66, no. 42 (17 October 1988): 5; Brad Stone, "How AIDS Has Changed FDA," *FDA Consumer* 24, no. 1 (February 1990): 14.

5 James Scheuer, "The FDA: Too Slow," *New York Times*, 22 May 1980, A35; Richert, *Conservatism, Consumer Choice, and the Food and Drug Administration*, 68.

6 Richert, *Conservatism, Consumer Choice, and the Food and Drug Administration*, 62.

7 Testimony of Louis Lasagna, M.D. on Drug Regulation Reform Act of 1978 before the Subcommittee on Health and Scientific Research and Committee on Human Resources (Rochester, NY: The Center for the Study of Drug Development, 12 April 1978), 2.

8 Committee on Science and Technology, *Drug Lag*, 97th Congress, 1st Session, 16 September 1981, 2.

9 Richert, *Conservatism, Consumer Choice, and the Food and Drug Administration*, 62–3.

10 *FDA and the 96th Congress* (Washington, DC: Food and Drug Administration, 1980), 135–6.

11 Anthony A. Celeste and Arthur N. Levine, "The Mission and the Institution: Ever Changing Yet Eternally the Same," in Pines, ed., *FDA*, 71–98.

12 Baer, *Biomedicine and Alternative Healing Systems in America*, 106–9; De Spain, *The Little Cyanide Cookbook*; Griffin, *World without Cancer*; Markle and Peterson, *Politics, Science, and Cancer*.

13 Holden, "Laetrile," 984.

14 "Laetrile Crackdown," *Time* 107, no. 24 (7 June 1976): 84. See also "Challenging the Apricot-Pit Gang," *Time* 110, no. 4 (25 July 1977).

15 Patterson, *The Dread Disease*, ix.

16 Ibid.

17 Moss, *The Cancer Industry*, 147.

18 Carpenter, *Reputation and Power*, 412.

19 Quoted in Young, *American Health Quackery*, 216.

20 Young, *The Medical Messiahs*, 453. See also Kittler, *Laetrile*.

21 Young, *American Health Quackery*, 242–3.

22 Richardson and Griffin, *Laetrile Case Histories*.

23 Bradford and Culbert, "The Laetrile Phenomenon," 179–80.

24 Cohen, "Michael L. Culbert," 16.

25 Ibid.

26 Holden, "Laetrile," 982–3; Culbert, *Vitamin B-17*; Culbert, *Freedom from Cancer*.

27 Grossman, "The Rise of the Empowered Consumer," 36.

28 See "Beating Autism: How I Saved My Son," *US Weekly*, 27 October 2008, and Amy Elisa Keith, "Fighting Autism with My Son," *People*, 4 June 2007, http://people.com/archive/fighting-autism-with-my-son-vol-67-no-22/. McCarthy has also written a number of books, including McCarthy, *Louder than Words: A Mother's Journey in Healing Autism* (New York: Dutton, 2007); McCarthy, *Mother Warriors: A Nation of Parents Healing Autism against All Odds* (New York: Dutton, 2009); McCarthy and Jerry Kartinzel, *Healing and Preventing Autism: A Complete Guide* (New York: Dutton, 2010). See also Offit's *Autism's False Prophets* and *Deadly Choices*.

29 Landau, review of *World without Cancer*, 696.

30 Crippen and Veatch, "Laetrile," 18.

31 Relman, "Laetrilomania," 215–16; Lewis Grossman, "FDA and the Rise of the Empowered Patient," in Cohen and Lynch, eds., *FDA in the 21st Century*, 65–6.

32 Walsh, "Laetrile Tops FDA's Most Unwanted List," 158–9.

33 US Food and Drug Administration, FDA *Quarterly Activities Report*, FY 1978, 1st Quarter (Washington, DC, 1975), 53.

34 Carpenter, *Reputation and Power*, 416; Nightingale, "Laetrile," 336.

35 Grossman, "FDA and the Rise of the Empowered Patient," 66.

36 Schwantes, *In Mountain Shadows*, 242; Representative Steven D. Symms, interview, "Legalize Laetrile as a Cancer Drug?" *U.S. News and World Report* 82 (13 June 1977): 51; Grossman, "FDA and the Rise of the Empowered Patient," 66.

37 Dennis F. Thompson, "Paternalism in Medicine, Law, and Public Policy," in Callahan and Bok, eds., *Ethics Teaching in Higher Education*, 267.

38 "Bill Could Legalize Marijuana," *Spokane Daily Chronicle*, 7 July 1977, 5.

39 Reagan et al., *Reagan, In His Own Hand*, 298.

40 Schwantes, *In Mountain Shadows*, 242; Carpenter, *Reputation and Power*, 529.

41 Lawrence Altman, "Some States Going beyond Laetrile to Legalize Unlicensed Substances," *New York Times*, 8 June 1977, A16.

42 Crippen and Veatch, "Laetrile," 18.

43 "Court Ruling on Laetrile Seen by F.D.A. as Curb," *New York Times*, 27 February 1980, A19.

44 "Challenging the Apricot-Pit Gang," *Time*, 64. See also Benjamin Wilson, "The Rise and Fall of Laetrile," accessed 11 October 2016, http://www.quackwatch.org/01QuackeryRelatedTopics/Cancer/laetrile.html.

45 Moertel, "A Trial of Laetrile Now," 218–19.

46 Wayne Pines, "Fighting Laetrile," in Pines, ed., FDA, 176–7.

47 "Laetrile Crackdown," *Time*, 84.

48 PDQ®, "PDQ Laetrile/Amygdalin." See also Relman, "Closing the Books on Laetrile," 236.

49 "Laetrile Flunks," *Time* 117, no. 19 (11 May 1981): 63.

50 Quoted in Moss, *The Cancer Industry*, 151.

51 National Cancer Institute, "Clinical Study of Laetrile in Cancer Patients, Investigators' Report: A Summary," 30 April 1981.

52 Sun, "Laetrile Brush Fire Is Out, Scientists Hope," 758.

53 Ibid., 758–9.

54 Ibid.

55 Eliot, *Steve McQueen*; Jackson et al., *The Intersection of Star Culture*, 14–16.

56 Bill Royce, "Steve McQueen Refutes Rumors about Cancer," *Boca Raton News*, 26 March 1980, 5C.

57 Jackson et al., *The Intersection of Star Culture*, 15.

58 Cohen, *Patients with Passports*; Colleen Walsh, "The Rise of Medical Tourism," *Harvard Gazette*, 16 October 2012, http://news.harvard.edu/gazette/story/2012/10/the-rise-of-medical-tourism/.

59 Barron Lerner, "McQueen's Legacy of Laetrile," *New York Times*, 15 November 2005 http://www.nytimes.com/2005/11/15/health/mcqueens-legacy-of-laetrile.html.

60 Ibid.

61 Kathy Mackay, "Steve McQueen, Stricken with Cancer, Seeks a Cure at a Controversial Mexican Clinic," *People* 14, no. 16 (20 October 1980), http://www.people.com/people/archive/article/0,,20077667,00.html.

62 Lerner, *When Illness Goes Public*.

63 Troetel, "Three Part Disharmony," 24.

64 Nightingale, "Laetrile," 333.

65 "Vitamin B17 Controversy: Poison or Cancer Treatment," *Dr. Axe: Food Is Medicine*, accessed 27 January 2017, https://draxe.com/vitamin-b17/.

66 "About Dr. Axe," *Dr. Axe: Food Is Medicine*, accessed 27 January 2017, https://draxe.com/about-dr-josh-axe/.

CHAPTER FOUR.

1 Rucker, "Views and Reviews"; "End the Ban on Psychoactive Drug Research," *Scientific American*, 1 February 2014, http://www. scientificamerican.com/article/end-the-ban-on-psychoactive-drug-research/; Sessa, "Turn On and Tune In," 10–12; James Randerson, "Lancet Calls for LSD in Labs," *The Guardian*, 14 April 2006, https://www.theguardian.com/science/2006/apr/14/medicalresearch. drugs.

2 Ibid.

3 Sessa Interview.

4 Ibid.

5 Ibid.

6 Bennet, "LSD," 1219–22. See also Sessa, *The Psychedelic Renaissance*.

7 Langlitz, *Neuropsychedelia*.

8 "Ralph Metzner on Acid & Culture," *High Times* 2 (1977–78): 32.

9 "End the Ban on Psychoactive Drug Research," *Scientific American*.

10 Hofmann, LSD.

11 Ibid, 18.

12 Ibid, 15–16.

13 See ibid., 42, and Dyck, *Psychedelic Psychiatry*.

14 Bennet, "LSD," 1219.

15 Michael Pollan, "The Trip Treatment: Research into Psychedelics, Shut Down for Decades, Is Now Yielding Exciting Results," *The New Yorker*, 9 February 2015, http://www.newyorker.com/ magazine/2015/02/09/trip-treatment.

16 For one example of the diversity, see Abramson, *The Use of LSD in Psychotherapy*.

17 For more on this, see Ellwood, *The Sixties Spiritual Awakening*. For discussions on the religious manifestations of the psychedelic movement and the spiritual use of LSD and psychedelics, see Kripal, *Esalen*, 125–30.

18 See Hoffer and Osmond, *The Hallucinogens*.

19 See Dyck and Bradford, "Peyote on the Prairies," 28–52. See also Wasson, *Soma*, and Furst, *Flesh of the Gods*.

20 Hoffer and Osmond, *The Hallucinogens*, 237–66. For another example, see Labate and Feeney, "Ayahuasca and the Process of Regulation in Brazil," 154–61.

21 Osmond, "A Review of the Clinical Effects of Psychotomimetic Agents," 418–34.

22 Hollingshead, "Some Issues in the Epidemiology of Schizophrenia," 6–7; Dixon, "Schizophrenia Controversy," 265.

23 Abram Hoffer, "Humphry Osmond: Countering Schizophrenia with Vitamins," *The Guardian*, 26 February 2004; Barber, *Psychedelic Revolutionaries*.

24 Peasley, "For Patients Having Coma Shock Therapy," 623–6.

25 Quoted in Dickinson, *The Two Psychiatries*, 123.

26 Gibson, "How ECT Works," 169; Kelly, "Fractures Complicate ECT," 98–9. See also Sadowsky, *Electroconvulsive Therapy in America*.

27 Dyck, "Land of the Living Skies with Diamonds," 53–4.

28 Mills, "Lessons from the Periphery," 186–9.

29 For a more recent meta-analysis of these results, see Krebs and Johansen, "Lysergic Acid Diethylamide (LSD) for Alcoholism," 994–1002.

30 See, for example, Dyck, "Hitting Highs at Rock Bottom," 313–30; Mangini, "Treatment of Alcoholism Using Psychedelic Drugs," 381–418.

31 Healy, *The Creation of Psychopharmacology*, 41.

32 Ibid.

33 For more on Kesey, see Dodgson, *It's All a Kind of Magic*.

34 Greenfield, *Timothy Leary*.

35 Pamphlet, "Castalia Foundation: Experiential Workshops," MS Laing GM139, R.D. Laing Collection, Special Collections, University of Glasgow.

36 Kesey, *One Flew Over the Cuckoo's Nest*.

37 Erika Dyck, "The Psychedelic Sixties in North America: Drugs and Identity," in Campbell et al., eds., *Debating Dissent*, 47–66. See Matthew Oram's work. Oram is currently working on a book for Johns Hopkins University Press called *The Trials of Psychedelic Medicine: LSD Psychotherapy in the United States*.

38 Willliam Hynes, "Mapping the Characteristics of Mythic Tricksters: A Heuristic Guide," in Hynes and Doty, eds., *Mythical Trickster Figures*, 33–45. See Radin, *The Trickster*, 195–211.

39 Burston, *The Crucible of Experience*; Thompson, *The Legacy of R. D. Laing*; Chitra Ramaswamy, "Return to Oz: The Most Controversial Magazine of the 60s Goes Online," *The Guardian*, 6 March 2016, https://www.theguardian.com/media/shortcuts/2016/mar/06/return-oz-most-controversial-magazine-60s-goes-online.

40 "Letter between R.D. Laing and Gunter Weil," 20 January 1965, GW44, MS Laing GW4-52, Laing Collection, Special Collections, University of Glasgow.

41 "Comments on a Provisional Draft 'LYCERGIC ACID DIETHYLAMIDE,'" MS Laing GM139, R.D. Laing Collection, Special Collections, University of Glasgow.

42 Ibid.

43 McWilliams, "Unsung Partner Against Crime," 207–36; James Sterba, "The Politics of Pot," *Esquire* 61 (August 1968): 118–19.

44 Paul Lowinger, "Psychiatrists, Marihuana, and the Law: A Survey," paper presented at the American Orthopsychiatric Association annual meeting, San Francisco, 23–26 March 1970; Barron et al., "A Clinical Examination of Chronic LSD Use in the Community," 69–79. See also Lowinger and Polakoff, "Do Medical Students 'Turn On'?" 185–8.

45 Paul Lowinger, "The Doctor as Political Activist: A Progress Report," paper presented at the Conference on Radicals in the Professions, Ann Arbor, MI, 14–16 July 1967: ARBML, WL Ms Coll. 592, Box 63, Folder 806.

46 Ibid.

47 William Braden, "LSD and the Press," in Aaronson and Osmond, eds., *Psychedelics*, 400–17.

48 For these and other examples, see Dyck, *Psychedelic Psychiatry*, ch. five.

49 Gallagher, "Tripped Out," 162. Also Benshoff, "The Short-Lived Life," 29–44, which elucidates the "LSD Film" genre.

50 Siff, *Acid Hype*, 187.

51 B. Humphry Osmond to Jonathan Cole, Chief, Psychopharmacology Service Centre, National Institute of Health, 9 February 1967, A207, XVIII, 20, Provincial Archives of Saskatchewan, Regina, Saskatchewan.

52 Oram, "Efficacy and Enlightenment," 221–50.

53 As quoted in Jonnes, *Hep-Cats, Narcs, and Pipe Dreams*, 232.

54 Erika Dyck, "'Just Say Know': Criminalizing LSD and the Politics of Psychedelic Expertise, 1961–68," in Montigny, ed., *The Real Dope*, 169–96.

55 Lisa Bieberman, "The Psychedelic Experience," *The New Republic*, 5 August 1967, 17–18.

56 For examples of these studies, see Aaronson and Osmond, *Psychedelics*. Chapter titles indicate this shift in tone, and include:

"Mescaline: On Being Mad"; "LSD: Who Am I, and So What If I Am?"; "Yage: Yage in the Valley of Fire"; "Mushrooms and the Mind"; etc.

57 Bieberman, "The Psychedelic Experience," 18.

58 Stevens, *Storming Heaven.*

59 Chris Ayres and Penny Wark, "Turn On, Tune In, Feel Better: Psychedelic Drugs Including LSD, Demonised since the 1960s, Are Back on the Research Agenda," *The Times*, 27 April 2010, 8.

60 Andrew M. Brown, "Psychedelic Revival: Mind-Bending Drugs Are Making a Comeback – In the Field of Psychiatry," *The Spectator*, 18 August 2012, 18–19.

61 Sessa Interview.

62 Kuzmarov, "From Counter-Insurgency to Narco-Insurgency"; Gorman, "'War on Drugs' Continues," 307; Schrag, "A Quagmire for Our Time," 286–98.

63 Emerson et al., "History and Future," 27–8.

64 Musto and Korsmeyer, *The Quest for Drug Control.*

65 Horgan, "The Electric Kool-Aid Clinical Trial," 36–40; Morris, "Research on Psychedelics," 1491–2. See also Emerson et al., "History and Future," 28.

66 Grof is the author of *Realms of the Human Unconscious.*

67 Emerson et al., "History and Future," 28.

68 For a fuller account of radical mental health therapy in the 1960s and 1970s, see Richert, "'Therapy Means Change, Not Peanut Butter.'"

69 Brown, "Research on Psychedelics," 23–4.

70 Gary Stix, "Return of a Problem Child," *Scientific American*, October 2009, 8.

71 Langlitz, *Neuropsychedelia*, 13.

72 Smith et al., "From Hofmann to the Haight Ashbury," 9–10; Shrubb, "The Magical Mystery Cure," 10. As of this writing, Gasser's MAPS-funded project has not published its findings in a peer-reviewed scientific journal.

73 Langlitz, *Neuropsychedelia*, 51.

74 Vollenweider and Kometer, "The Neurobiology of Psychedelic Drugs," 642–8.

75 Ibid., 648.

76 Smith et al., "From Hofmann to Haight Ashbury," 6.

77 Quoted in Langlitz, *Neuropsychedelia*, 79.

78 Winkler and Csémy, "Self-Experimentations with Psychedelics," 16.

79 Vollenweider and Kometer, "The Neurobiology of Psychedelic Drugs," 648.

80 Miles O'Brien, "Why Psychedelic Drugs Are Having a Medical Renaissance," PBS *Newshour*, 25 January 2017, http://www.pbs.org/newshour/bb/psychedelic-drugs-medical-renaissance/.

CHAPTER FIVE

1 Martel, *Not This Time*; Montigny, ed., *The Real Dope*; Lee, *Smoke Signals*. In the UK, Mills has produced books that showcase the global and British history of cannabis. See his *Cannabis Britannica* and *Cannabis Nation*.

2 John Burns, "Osgood Law Dean Heads Federal Drug Investigation," *Globe and Mail*, 4 June 1969, A1.

3 Ibid.

4 Brecher, *Licit and Illicit Drugs*.

5 Ian McLeod, "Public Hearings, Two Trudeaus and 'Reefer Madness' Fear-Mongering: The Long War over Marijuana Legalization," *National Post*, 26 December 2015, http://news.nationalpost.com/news/canada/canadian-politics/public-hearings-two-trudeaus-and-decades-of-reefer-madness-fear-mongering-the-long-war-over-the-legalization-of-marijuana; Lee, *Smoke Signals*, 131; Kate Allen, "Why Canada Banned Pot (Science Had Nothing to Do with It)," *Toronto Star*, 1 December 2013, https://www.thestar.com/news/canada/2013/12/01/why_canada_banned_pot_ science_had_ nothing_to_do_with_it.html.

6 Allen, "Why Canada Banned Pot."

7 "Le Dain Report on Drugs Divides Cabinet," CBC *Radio*, 21 June 1970, http://www.cbc.ca/archives/entry/ledain-report-on-drugs-divides-cabinet.

8 Library of Parliament, House of Commons Debates, 32nd Parliament, 1st Session: Vol. 12. Speech by Mr Mel Gass (Malpeque) December 11, 1981: 13998.

9 Ibid.

10 Library of Parliament, House of Commons Debates, 32nd Parliament, 1st Session: Vol. 9. Speech by Mr Dan McKenzie (Winnipeg-Assiniboine) May 15, 1981: 9651.

11 Caroline Barghout, "Medical Marijuana Patients Using Health Canada Licenses to Sell Pot Legally," CBC *News*, 30 September 2016,

http://www.cbc.ca/news/canada/manitoba/medical-marijuana-licences-1.3784620.

12 Trinh Theresa Do, "Medical Marijuana Legal in All Forms, Supreme Court Rules," CBC News, 11 June 2015, http://www.cbc.ca/news/politics/medical-marijuana-legal-in-all-forms-supreme-court-rules-1.3109148.

13 Greg Engel, "No Need to Reinvent the Wheel on Cannabis," National Post, 26 October 2015, http://news.nationalpost.com/full-comment/greg-engel-no-need-to-reinvent-the-wheel-on-cannabis.

14 "First Health Canada Approved Medical Cannabis Clinical Trial Starts Patient Recruitment," NewsWire, 23 June 2015, http://www.newswire.ca/news-releases/first-health-canada-approved-medical-cannabis-clinical-trial-starts-patient-recruitment-518025911.html; Peter Koven and David Pett, "Marijuana Firms Tweed and Bedrocan to Merge to Create Dominant Canadian Player," National Post, 24 June 2015, http://business.financialpost.com/investing/marijuana-firms-tweed-and-bedrocan-to-merge-to-create-dominant-canadian-player?__lsa=dbb5-6b49.

15 Dan Levin, "As Canada Moves to Legalize Marijuana, Shop Owners Ask: Why Wait?" New York Times, 16 August 2016, A6.

16 Daniel LeBlanc, "Marijuana Task Force Faces 'Fascinating Journey' in Crafting Legal Framework," The Globe and Mail, 18 July 2016, http://www.theglobeandmail.com/news/politics/marijuana-task-force-faces-fascinating-journey-in-crafting-legal-framework/article30973622/.

17 Cady Lang, "Justin Trudeau Makes a Surprising Case for Legalizing Marijuana," Time, 10 June 2016, http://time.com/4364344/justin-trudeau-marijuana-weed-legal/.

18 Levin, "Canada Moves to Legalize Marijuana."

19 Lucas Richert, "Clarify Pot Policy for Veterans," Saskatoon StarPhoenix, 6 May 2016, http://thestarphoenix.com/opinion/letters/0506-edit-richert-view; Catherine Cullen, "As Veterans' Pot Prescriptions Rise Tenfold in 2 Years, Ottawa Asks Questions," CBC News, 14 March 2016, http://www.cbc.ca/news/politics/veterans-marijuana-bill-forces-1.3487516.

20 Catherine Cullen, "Veterans Advocate Says Let Doctors Decide on Medical Marijuana," CBC News, 30 April 2016, http://www.cbc.ca/news/politics/veterans-doctors-medical-marijuana-1.3555235.

21 Levin, "Canada Moves to Legalize Marijuana."

22 "Legalising Pot in Canada," *The Economist*, 19 December 2015.
23 Lucas Richert, "Pot Problems Have a Familiar Ring," *Saskatoon StarPhoenix*, 18 September 2015, http://thestarphoenix.com/news/local-news/pot-problems-have-familiar-ring.
24 Ibid.
25 Ibid.
26 Dave Deibert, "Saskatoon Police Insist 'Charges Were Appropriate' against Marijuana Compassion Club," *Saskatoon StarPhoenix*, 3 November 2015, http://thestarphoenix.com/news/local-news/saskatoon-police-insist-charges-were-appropriate-against-marijuana-compassion-club.
27 Kathy Fitzpatrick, "Saskatoon Top Place in Canada to Be Charged for Marijuana Possession," cbc *News*, 30 September 2015, http://www.cbc.ca/news/canada/saskatoon/saskatoon-top-place-in-canada-to-be-charged-for-marijuana-possession-1.3249579; "Eloise Opheim letter to Otto Moulton," 20 June 1985, Robert J. Dole Senate Papers-Legislative Relations, 1969–1996, Series 6, Box 676, Folder 2, Robert J. Dole Archive and Special Collections, University of Kansas, Lawrence, Kansas.
28 Murray Opdahl, "Medical Cannabis: The Canadian Physicians' Perspective," *ActiveHistory.ca*, 30 March 2016, http://activehistory.ca/2016/03/medical-cannabis-the-canadian-physicians-perspective/.
29 Ibid.
30 Canadian Medical Association, "cma Policy" and "Statement on Health Canada's Proposed Changes to Medical Marijuana Regulations."
31 The College of Family Physicians of Canada, "Statement on Health Canada's Proposed Changes to Medical Marijuana Regulations."
32 College of Physicians and Surgeons of British Columbia, "Professional Standards and Guidelines." See also Ware et al., "Smoked Cannabis for Chronic Neuropathic Pain," E694–701; Ware et al., "Cannabis for the Management of Pain," 1233–42; College of Physicians and Surgeons of Saskatchewan, "Prescribing Medical Marihuana"; Lynch and Campbell, "Cannabinoids for Treatment of Chronic Non-cancer Pain," 735–44.
33 Vann R. Newkirk II, "What Can't Medical Marijuana Do?" *The Atlantic*, July 2016, accessed 14 October 2016, http://www.theatlantic.com/politics/archive/2016/07/medical-marijuana-costs-elderly-health/491306/.
34 Miller, "The Cannabis Conundrum," 17165.

35   Fischer et al., "Medical Marijuana Programs," 15–19.

36   Ibid.

37   Bill Curry and Steven Chase, "Trudeau Reignites Legalization Debate with Admission to Smoking Marijuana," *Globe and Mail*, 22 August 2013, http://www.theglobeandmail.com/news/politics/justin-trudeau-details-history-with-marijuana-smoked-pot-as-recently-as-three-years-ago/article13911495/.

38   Althia Raj, "Justin Trudeau Smoked Marijuana After Becoming MP," *Huffington Post*, 22 August 2013, http://www.huffingtonpost.ca/2013/08/22/justin-trudeau-marijuana-mp_n_3792208.html.

39   Ibid.

40   Robin Mackay and Karin Phillips, *The Legal Regulation of Marijuana in Canada and Selected Other Countries* (Ottawa: Library of Parliament, 2016), accessed 18 January 2017, http://publications.gc.ca/collections/collection_2016/bdp-lop/bp/YM32-2-2016-94-eng.pdf, 6, 10; Task Force on Marijuana Legalization and Regulation, *Toward the Legalization, Regulation and Restriction of Access to Marijuana: Discussion Paper* (Ottawa: Government of Canada, 2016), accessed 18 January 2017, http://publications.gc.ca/collections/collection_2016/jus/J11-2016-1-eng.pdf, 3.

41   Porath-Waller et al., *What Canadian Youth Think about Cannabis*, 21.

42   Ibid., 2, 21–2.

43   Ibid., 36.

44   Task Force, *Toward Legalization*, 3.

45   For example, see MP and physician Dr Kellie Leitch's opposition, cited in Evan Dyer, "Tory Leadership Race Sparks Issue of Marijuana Legalization," CBC *News*, 16 April 2016, http://www.cbc.ca/news/politics/marijuana-leadership-bernier-leitch-ambrose-1.3527691. See also Fischer et al., "Cannabis Use in Canada," 101–3.

46   Canada, Parliament, House of Commons, Standing Committee on Health, *Marijuana's Health Risks and Harms: Report of the Standing Committee on Health* (Ottawa: Standing Committee on Health, 2014), accessed 18 January 2017, http://www.parl.gc.ca/content/hoc/Committee/412/HESA/Reports/RP6728826/hesarp06/hesarp06-e.pdf, 17.

47   Ibid.

48   Kahan et al., "Prescribing Smoked Cannabis for Chronic Noncancer Pain," 1083–90.

49 Health Canada, *Information for Health Care Professionals: Cannabis (Marihuana, Marijuana) and Cannabinoids* (Ottawa: Health Canada, 2013), accessed 18 January 2017, http://publications.gc.ca/collections/collection_2016/sc-hc/H129-19-2013-eng.pdf, ii.

50 Health Canada, *Consumer Information–Cannabis (Marihuana, Marijuana)* (Ottawa: Health Canada, 2016), accessed 18 January 2017, http://publications.gc.ca/collections/collection_2016/sc-hc/H129-20-2016-eng.pdf, 1.

51 Standing Committee on Health, *Marijuana's Health Risks*, 4.

52 Ibid., 7, 9.

53 Hill, "Perspective," S14.

54 See Kalant's "A Critique of Cannabis Legalization Proposals in Canada," 5–10, and "Cannabis Control Policy," 538–40.

55 Sznitman and Zolotov, "Cannabis for Therapeutic Purposes," 20–9.

56 Lake et al., "Prescribing Medical Cannabis in Canada," E328.

57 Anindya Sen, *Joint Venture: A Blueprint for Federal and Provincial Marijuana Policy* (Toronto: C.D. Howe Institute, 2016), 3.

58 Campos et al., "Multiple Mechanisms," 3364; Pajevic et al., "Do Cannabis and Cannabinoids Have a Psychofarmalogically Therapeutic Effect?" 1068.

59 Cohen, "Cannabinoids for Chronic Pain," 167–8.

60 Ibid.

61 George Skelton, "Marijuana Is Legal in California. Now Politicians and Pot Pushers Need to Help Keep It out of Kids' Hands," *Los Angeles Times*, 5 January 2017, http://www.latimes.com/politics/la-pol-sac-skelton-marijuana-legalization-teens-20170105-story.html.

62 Page and Ware, "Perspective," S9.

63 Room, "Cannabis Legalization and Public Health," 358–9; Spithoff et al., "Cannabis Legalization," 1211–16.

64 Fischer et al., "Realistically Furthering the Goals of Public Health," 11–16; Uchtenhagen, "Some Critical Issues in Cannabis Policy Reform," 356–8.

65 Lough, "Growing the Evidence Base for Medical Cannabis," 955–6.

66 Allison Tierney, "Canadians and Americans Spent 72$ Billion on Weed Last Year," *Vice*, 20 January 2017, https://www.vice.com/en_ca/article/canadians-and-americans-spent-dollar72-billion-on-weed-last-year.

67 See Lenton, "New Regulated Markets for Recreational Cannabis," 354–5.

68 Reid Southwick, "Investors Dive into Marijuana Stocks, Raising Concerns about Green Bubble," *Calgary Herald*, 27 January 2017, http://calgaryherald.com/business/local-business/investors-dive-into-marijuana-stocks-raising-concerns-about-green-bubble.

69 Sadaf Ahsan, "Snoop Dogg Signs Exclusive Deal with Canadian Marijuana Producer," *National Post*, 12 February 2016, http://news.nationalpost.com/arts/celebrity/snoop-dogg-signs-exclusive-deal-with-canadian-marijuana-producer.

70 Centre for Addiction and Mental Health, "Cannabis Policy Framework," 8.

71 Ibid., 16.

72 Ibid., 15.

73 Macleod and Hickman, "How Ideology Shapes the Evidence and the Policy," 1326–30.

74 Macleod and Hickman, "Response to Commentaries," 1337–9.

75 This story is detailed in Allan M. Brandt, *The Cigarette Century*.

76 Gundle et al., "'To Prove This Is the Industry's Best Hope,'" 974–83.

77 See Barry et al., "Waiting for the Opportune Moment," 207.

78 Henry et al., "Comparing Cannabis With Tobacco," 942–3; Iversen, "Comparing Cannabis with Tobacco," 165; Sidney, "Comparing Cannabis With Tobacco – Again," 635–6.

79 Committee on the Health Effects of Marijuana, *The Health Effects of Cannabis and Cannabinoids*, 5-1.

CHAPTER SIX

1 Kushner, "The Other War on Drugs," 49–70; Committee on Government Operations, FDA*'s Regulation of Zomax*, 98th Congress, 1st Session, 26 and 27 April 1983, 443; Healy, *Let Them Eat Prozac*.

2 Avorn, *Powerful Medicines*, 222–4.

3 Robert Pear, "Bush Hints at Policy Shifts on Canadian Drug Imports," *New York Times*, 12 October 2004, http://www.nytimes.com/2004/10/12/politics/campaign/bush-hints-at-policy-shift-on-canadian-drug-imports.html?_r=0.

4 I use the phrase deliberately. See Malleck, *When Good Drugs Go Bad*, and Giacomini et al., "When Good Drugs Go Bad," 975–7.

5 Kevin Libin, "EpiPen's Mylan and Martin Shkreli Rip Off Patients with the Help of Government, not Capitalism," *Financial Post*, 29 August 2016, http://business.financialpost.com/fp-comment/kevin-libin-epipens-mylan-and-martin-shkreli-rip-off-patients-with-the-help-of-government-not-capitalism; McCarthy, "Epinephrine Pen Maker Offers Discount after Alleged Price Hiking"; Bethany McLean, "Everything You Know about Martin Shkreli Is Wrong – Or Is It?" *Vanity Fair*, February 2016, accessed 14 October 2016, http://www.vanityfair.com/news/2015/12/martin-shkreli-pharmaceuticals-ceo-interview.

6 "HHS Secretary Thompson Reviews US Drug Re-import Bill, to Dismay of PHRMA," *The Pharma Letter*, 9 March 2001, http://www.thepharmaletter.com/article/hhs-sec-thompson-reviews-us-drug-re-import-bill-to-dismay-of-phrma.

7 Cohen, "Pushing the Borders," 16; Brett J. Skinner, "Prescription Piracy: The Black Market in Foreign Drugs Will Not Reduce U.S. Healthcare Costs," in Graham, ed., *What States Can Do to Reform Health Care*, 83–97.

8 Halberstam, *War in a Time of Peace*, 298.

9 Ibid.

10 Lawler and Stone, "FDA," 1038–41.

11 Quoted in Greg Anrig, "Who Strangled the FDA?" *The American Prospect*, 12 December 2007, http://prospect.org/article/who-strangled-fda.

12 Quoted in Hilts, *Protecting America's Health*, 313.

13 Ibid.

14 "FDA in 1996: Twice as NCE," 6.

15 Hilts, *Protecting America's Health*, 311.

16 Robert Dreyfuss, "Popping Contributions: The New Battle for the FDA," *The American Prospect* 33 (July/August 1997): 58.

17 Ibid.

18 Dickinson, "Gingrich Plan for the FDA Leaves Questions," 10.

19 Hilts, *Protecting America's Health*, 313.

20 Richert, *Conservatism, Consumer Choice, and the Food and Drug Administration*.

21 Angell, *The Truth about Drug Companies*; Fukuyama, *Our Posthuman Future*; Healy, *Mania*; Watters, *Crazy Like Us*.

22 Greene, *Prescribing by Numbers*; Tobbell, "'Who's Winning the Human Race?'" 429–73; Dyck, *Psychedelic Psychiatry*; Herzberg,

Happy Pills in America; Kuzmarov, *The Myth of the Addicted Army*; Schneider, *Smack*.

23 Bhosle and Balkrishnan, "Drug Reimportation Practices in the United States," 41–6; Geoffrey Colvin, "We Hate BigPharma, but We Sure Love Drugs," *Fortune*, 27 December 2004, http://archive. fortune.com/magazines/fortune/fortune_archive/2004/12/27/ 8217957/index.htm; Finkelstein and Temin, *Reasonable RX*.

24 Shepherd, "Drug Importation," 1288–91.

25 Joel Baglole, "Health Costs/Prevention – Getting the Gray Out: Canadian and U.S. Regulators Are Looking to Impose Order on the Sale of Cheap Online Drugs," *Wall Street Journal*, 11 February 2003, R6.

26 Bhosle and Balkrishnan, "Drug Reimportation Practices in the United States," 41–6; Geoff Dyer, "Drugs Group Gets Tough on Canada," *Financial Times*, 14 January 2003, 2; Philip Elliot, "McCain Calls for Drug Reimportation," *Washington Post*, 17 November 2007, http://www.washingtonpost.com/wp-dyn/content/ article/2007/11/17/AR2007111700850.html.

27 Hawthorne, *Inside the* FDA.

28 Bhosle and Balkrishnan, "Drug Reimportation Practices in the United States," 41–6; Baglole, "Health Costs/Prevention"; Saatsoglou, "Pharmaceutical Reimportation," 7–9.

29 Herzberg, *Happy Pills in America*, 127 (italics mine).

30 Ibid.

31 Carpenter, *Reputation and Power*; Daemmrich, *Pharmacopolitics*; Scroop, "A Faded Passion?" 1–17; John Swann, "Pharmaceutical Regulation Before and After the Food Drugs and Cosmetics Act," in Berry and Martin, eds., *The Pharmaceutical Regulatory Process*, 1–29.

32 Avorn, *Powerful Medicines*, 44; Carpenter, *Reputation and Power*, 188–91.

33 Miller and Henderson, "The FDA's Risky Risk-Aversion," 8–11.

34 Lybecker, "Economics of Reimportation," 10–14.

35 US Congress, House of Representatives, Testimony of William K. Hubbard, Associate Commissioner for Policy, Planning and Legislation, *The Importation of Drugs into the United States*, Hearings Before the Committee on Energy and Commerce, 107th Congress, 25 July 2002.

36 Nina Owcharenko, "Debunking the Myths of Drug Importation," *Heritage Foundation*, 20 July 2004, http://www.heritage.org/

research/reports/2004/07/debunking-the-myths-of-drug-importation; Congressional Budget Office, "Would Prescription Drug Importation Reduce U.S. Drug Spending?" *CBO: Economic and Budget Issue Brief*, 29 April 2004, https://www.cbo.gov/sites/default/files/108th-congress-2003-2004/reports/04-29-prescriptiondrugs.pdf; "FDA Crackdown on Illegal Products," *FDA Consumer* 38, no. 2 (2004): 36–7.

37 Rob Stein, "Ailing FDA May Need a Major Overhaul, Officials and Groups Say," *Washington Post*, 26 November 2008, A02.

38 Shepherd, "Drug Importation," 1289.

39 Robert Pear, "In a Turnaround, White House Kills Drug-Import Plan," *New York Times*, 27 December 2000, http://www.nytimes.com/2000/12/27/us/in-a-turnaround-white-house-kills-drug-import-plan.html; Donna Vogt, "Food and Drug Administration: Selected Funding and Policy Issues," in Hickman, ed., *The Food and Drug Administration*, 49–55.

40 Michele Meadows, "Imported Drugs Raise Safety Concerns," *FDA Consumer* 36, no. 5 (2002): 20.

41 Peter Rost, "Medicines without Borders," *New York Times*, 30 October 2004, http://www.nytimes.com/2004/10/30/opinion/medicines-without-borders.html.

42 Ibid.; Pear, "Bush Hints at Policy Shifts on Canadian Drug Imports."

43 Avorn, *Powerful Medicines*, 222.

44 Hawthorne, ed., *Inside the FDA*, 216; Owcharenko, "Debunking the Myths of Drug Reimportation," 3; Sarah Lueck, "FDA Defends Tougher Stance on Drug Imports," *Wall Street Journal*, 4 April 2003, A6; John Mack, "Drug Importation Crisis: Terror Politics to the Rescue!" *Pharma Marketing News* 3, no. 8 (2004), http://www.news.pharma-mkting.com/pmn38-oped.html.

45 US Congress, House of Representatives, Testimony of William K. Hubbard, Associate Commissioner for Policy, Planning and Legislation, Hearing Before the Committee on Commerce, Science and Transportation, 107th Congress, 5 September 2001; US Congress, House of Representatives, Testimony of William K. Hubbard, *The Importation of Drugs into the United States*, 25 July 2002; US Congress, Senate, Testimony of William K. Hubbard, Associate Commissioner for Policy, Planning and Legislation, *The Importation of Drugs into the United States*, Hearings Before the Special Committee on Aging, 107th Congress, 9 June 2002; US Congress, Senate, Testimony of William K. Hubbard and John M.

Taylor, *A System Overwhelmed: The Avalanche of Imported, Counterfeit and Unapproved Drugs in the U.S.*, Hearings Before the Committee on Governmental Affairs, 108th Congress, 24 June 2003; US Congress, House of Representatives, Testimony of William K. Hubbard, Associate Commissioner for Policy, Planning and Legislation, *Canadian Prescription Drug Reimportation: Is There a Safety Issue?* Hearings Before the Committee on Government Reform and Wellness, 108th Congress, 12 June 2003.

46 US Congress, Senate, Testimony of William K. Hubbard and John M. Taylor, *A System Overwhelmed*, 24 June 2003.

47 US Food and Drug Administration, Department of Health and Human Services, FDA *Counterfeit Drug Task Force Interim Report*, October 2003; Gardiner Harris, "Two Agencies to Fight Online Narcotic Sales," *New York Times*, 18 October 2003, http://www. nytimes.com/2003/10/18/business/two-agencies-to-fight-online-narcotics-sales.html?_r=0.

48 Thomas B. Edsall, "High Drug Prices Return as Issue That Stirs Voters; New Challenges for a Lobby Used to Spending," *Washington Post*, 15 October 2002, A8; Public Citizen's Congress Watch, "The Other Drug War 2003," 6–7.

49 Dyer, "Drug Group Gets Tough on Canada," 2; Mark Heinzl and Tamsin Carlisle, "Canadian Pharmacies Vs. Big Drug Makers; Online Retailers Vow to Fight Edicts Seeking to Clamp Down on Cheap Exports to the U.S.," *Wall Street Journal*, 12 August 2003, D4; Roger Parloff, "Pfizer Is Itching to Start a Drug War with Canada," *Fortune* 149, no. 6 (22 March 2004): 42.

50 Avorn, *Powerful Medicines*, 222–4.

51 Ibid.

52 Health Canada, "Buying Drugs over the Internet," November 2009, accessed 17 October 2016, http://publications.gc.ca/collections/ collection_2010/sc-hc/H13-7-68-2009-eng.pdf; Owcharenko, "Debunking the Myths of Drug Importation," 3; Ward, "Economic Policy Implications of Reimportation," 17–20.

53 Criminal Intelligence Service Canada, Public Safety Canada, "Counterfeit Pharmaceuticals in Canada," August 2006, accessed 17 March 2016, http://www.cisc.gc.ca/pharmaceuticals/documents/ counterfeit_pharmaceuticals_e.pdf, 2.

54 Hawthorne, *Inside the FDA*, 165.

55 Cohen, "Public Policy Implications," 14; Lueck, "FDA Defends Tougher Stance," A6.

56 Andrew Wilde Mathews, "Senate Panel Grills FDA Chief on Opposition to Drug Imports," *Wall Street Journal*, 12 March 2004, B4.

57 Stony Brook University, "Health Pulse of America," 5–25 November 2003, accessed 17 October 2016, http://www.stonybrook.edu/commcms/surveys/docs/Report%20Drug%20Importation_Nov%20 2003.pdf; The Kaiser Family Foundation/Harvard School of Public Health, "Medicare Prescription Drug Survey," 30 August 2003, http://www.kff.org/medicare/p0090303package.cfm; The Kaiser Family Foundation, "Health Care & the 2004 Elections: Prescription Drug Costs," 2 September 2004, http://www.kff.org/rxdrugs/7175.cfm.

58 Skinner, "Price Controls, Patents, and Cross-Border Internet Pharmacies," 29–34; Cohen, "Public Policy Implications," 16.

CHAPTER SEVEN

1 Jennifer Kerr, "Dr. Oz, Under Fire for Peddling 'Magic' Weight-Loss Aids, Promises to Publish List of Products that Actually Work," *National Post*, 18 June 2014, http://news.nationalpost.com/scene/dr-oz-under-fire-for-peddling-magic-weight-loss-aids-promises-to-publish-list-of-products-that-actually-work; Frank Bruni, "Hollywood Trumps Harvard," *New York Times*, 22 April 2015, http://www.nytimes.com/2015/04/22/opinion/frank-bruni-hollywood-trumps-harvard.html; "Dr. Oz Should Be Fired from Columbia for 'Promoting Quack Treatments': Top Physicians in Letter," *National Post*, 17 April 2015, http://news.nationalpost.com/health/dr-oz-should-be-fired-from-columbia-for-promoting-quack-treatments-top-physicians-in-letter?__lsa=e1c9-020e; see also Lucas Richert, "It's Time for Dr. Oz to Hit the Yellow Brick Road," *Alternet*, 8 May 2015, https://www.alternet.org/drugs/time-doctor-oz-hit-yellow-brick-road.

2 Elahe Izadi, "Dr. Oz Fires Back at His Critics: 'We Will Not Be Silenced,'" *Washington Post*, 23 April 2015, https://www.washingtonpost.com/news/to-your-health/wp/2015/04/23/dr-oz-goes-on-the-defensive-we-will-not-be-silenced/.

3 Park, "Historical Reflections on Diet, Exercise, and Obesity," 391–2.

4 Oliver, *Fat Politics*, and Finkelstein and Zuckerman, *The Fattening of America*.

5 Rizzolatti et al., "The Golden Beauty," e1201; Lasek and Gaulin, "Waist-Hip Ratio and Cognitive Ability," 26–34.

6 Mallory Schlossberg, "There's an Ugly Backlash against the Plus-Size Model Sports Illustrated Put on Its Cover," *Business Insider UK*, 27 February 2016, http://uk.businessinsider.com/ashley-graham-sports-illustrated-backlash-2016-2; Cole Delbyck, "Kesha Chews Up, Spits Out Body Shamer on Behalf of Everyone Who's Been Bullied," *Huffington Post*, 6 June 2016, http://www.huffingtonpost.com/entry/kesha-body-shaming-instagram_us_5752f024e4b0ed593f148e83.

7 Kevin Sack and Alicia Mundy, "A Dose of Denial," *Los Angeles Times*, 28 March 2004, http://www.latimes.com/la-na-ppa28mar28-1-htmlstory.html.

8 Ibid.

9 Lindsey Gruson, "A Controversy over Widely Sold Diet Pills," *New York Times*, 13 February 1982, http://www.nytimes.com/1982/02/13/style/a-controversy-over-widely-sold-diet-pills.html?pagewanted=all.

10 Sally E. Smith, "The Great Diet Deception," USA *Today* 123, no. 2596 (January 1995): 76.

11 Michael Lemonick and William Dowell, "The New Miracle Drug?" *Time* 148, no. 15 (23 September 1996): 62.

12 Schwartz, *Never Satisfied*; Stearns, *Fat History*, iii.

13 Historians have begun to examine health and fitness, as well as fatness, more closely. *The Canadian Bulletin of Medical History* 28, no. 2 (2011) recently devoted a special issue to sports medicine and fitness. See also Warsh, ed., *Gender, Health, and Popular Culture*, the recent launch of *The Fat Studies Journal* (2012), and the collaborative work on "fatness" by Wendy Mitchinson, Deborah McPhail, and Jenny Ellison.

14 "Medicine: Fletcherizing," *Time*, 17 September 1928; Pollan, *In Defense of Food*, 56–7.

15 Vester, "Regime Change," 39; Jackson, "The Art of Wishful Shrinking," 146–7.

16 Smith, *Eating History*, 247; Peters, *Diet and Health*.

17 Rowe and Silverstein, "The GDP Myth," 17–21.

18 Richard L. Cleland, Walter C. Gross, Laura D. Koss, Matthew Daynard, and Karen M. Muoio, "Weight-Loss Advertising: An Analysis of Current Trends," *A Report of the Staff of the Federal Trade Commission*, September 2002, accessed 18 October 2016,

http://news.findlaw.com/hdocs/docs/ftc/902weightlossadsrpt.pdf, 1–2.

19 "A Company That's Getting Fat Because America Wants to Be Thin," *Business Week*, 19 November 1984.

20 US Congress, Senate, Hearings Before the Select Committee on Nutrition and Human Needs, *National Nutrition Policy Study*, 1974, 93rd Congress, 2nd Session, June 1974.

21 US Congress, Senate, *Dietary Goals for the United States*, Prepared by the Staff of the Select Committee on Nutrition and Human Needs, 95th Congress, 1st Session, February 1977.

22 Marantz et al., "A Call for a Higher Standards," 234–5.

23 Lunde, "Health in the United States," 29–31; Barbara Schneeman, "Science and Public Health in the FDA's Regulation of Dietary Supplements," in Daemmrich and Radin, eds., *Perspectives on Risk and Regulation*, 115.

24 Collins, *Transforming America*, 152–5.

25 See Rees, "Characteristics, Content, and Significance," 317–22.

26 Batchelor and Stoddart, *The 1980s*, 81.

27 Glasser, "Fitness and the Postmodern Self," 181–2.

28 Kagan and Morse, "The Body Electronic," 165.

29 Carolyn McNurlen, "Popular Diets: Can You Stay on One and Stay Healthy?" *Better Homes and Gardens*, November 1984, 70.

30 Cleland et al., "Weight-Loss Advertising," viii–ix.

31 Ibid., 1–2.

32 Rowe and Silverstein, "The GDP Myth."

33 N.R. Kleinfield, "The Ever-Fatter Business of Thinness," *New York Times*, 7 September 1986, http://www.nytimes.com/1986/09/07/ business/the-ever-fatter-business-of-thinness.html?pagewanted=all.

34 "Starch Blockers Seized by FDA," *New York Times*, 1 October 1982, http://www.nytimes.com/1982/10/01/us/starch-blockers-seized-by-fda.html.

35 Kleinfield, "The Ever-Fatter Business of Thinness."

36 Ibid.

37 Milton Copulos, "The Controversy over Diet Drugs," *Consumer's Research*, May 1984, 16–19. Also see Lasagna, *Phenylpropanolomine*.

38 Lasagna, *Phenylpropanolamine*, 10–11.

39 Lake et al., "Phenylpropanolamine and Caffeine Use," 575–6.

40 "Nurses' Drug Alert: Diet Pills and Stroke," 1070; "Diet Pills: A
    Warning about Side Effects," *San Francisco Chronicle*, 15 September
    1983. Also see "A Company That's Getting Fat," *Business Week*, 17.

41 See Jenkins, *Decade of Nightmares*; Kalman, *Right Star Rising*;
    Killen, *1973 Nervous Breakdown*; Richert, "Surveying the
    Seventies"; Schulman, *The Seventies*.

42 See Abraham, *Science, Politics and the Pharmaceutical Industry*, 78;
    US Congress, House of Representatives, Committee on Science and
    Technology, *Drug Lag*, 97th Congress, 1st Session, 16 September
    1981, 2. See also US Department of Health, Education, and Welfare,
    Review Panel on New Drug Regulation: Final Report (Washington,
    DC: Department of Health, Education, and Welfare, 1977), 12–13.

43 Olson, "Substitution in Regulatory Agencies," 389; Burkholz, *The
    FDA*, 1–20; Fuchs and Anderson, "The Institutionalization of Cost-
    Benefit Analysis," 29–30; Richert, "Pills, Policy Making and
    Perceptions," 41–63.

44 Lowe, "Pharmaceutical Regulatory Policy," 504–9.

45 Ibid.

46 Philip J. Hilts, "Ailing Agency – The FDA and Safety: A Guardian of
    U.S. Health Is Under Stress," *New York Times*, 4 December 1989,
    A1.

47 James S. Benson, "State of the Food and Drug Administration,"
    speech, 18 May 1990, http://www.fda.gov/NewsEvents/Speeches/
    ucm107156.htm.

48 US Congress, Senate, Senate Republican Policy Committee,
    Legislative Notice: S.1082 – The FDA Revitalization Act, Number 13,
    30 April 2007; Quon, "Decisions at Scientific Agencies," 10–15.

49 Bill Grigg, "Memo," *Health and Human Services (HHS) News*, 25
    February 1982, 1.

50 Gruson, "A Controversy over Widely Sold Diet Pills."

51 "Diet Pills: A Warning about Side Effects," *San Francisco Chronicle*,
    15 September 1983.

52 Jane Brody, "Pills to Aid the Dieter: How Safe Are They?" *New York
    Times*, 9 November 1983, C1.

53 Michael Waldholz, "Drug in Several Diet Products May Cause Some
    Nervous Reactions, Researcher Says," *Wall Street Journal*, 13
    February 1981, 8.

54 Grigg, "Memo," 1.

55 US Congress, House of Representatives, House Select Committee on
    Aging, "Diet Pills," 98th Congress, 1st Session, 1983; "Congress

Considers Safety of Diet Aids," *American Pharmacy* 23, no. 9 (1983): 448.

56 Ibid.

57 "Congress Considers Safety of Diet Aids," *American Pharmacy*, 448.

58 Ibid.

59 Appleson, "Agencies Probe Safety," 1558. See also "Court Halts Misleading Diet Pill Advertisements," *Vegetarian Times* 72 (August 1983): 9.

60 Ibid.

61 Ibid.

62 Ibid.

63 Dean Siegal, "Medical Researchers Examine PPA," *News From Thompson Medical Company*, 12 June 1984, 26–30.

64 *The MacNeil/Lehrer Newshour*, "PPA," PBS, 11 June 1984.

65 Ibid.

66 Ibid.

67 Ibid.

68 "A Company That's Getting Fat," *Business Week*, 17.

69 Kleinfield, "The Ever-Fatter Business of Thinness."

70 Ibid.

71 Milton Copulos, "The Controversy over Diet Drugs," *Consumer's Research*, May 1984, 16–19.

72 Ibid.

73 Jeff Gerth and Sheryl Gay Stolberg, "Another Part of the Battle: Keeping a Drug on the Shelves of Stores," *New York Times*, 13 December 2000, 8. See also Morgan, *Phenylpropanolamine*.

74 Morgan was still publishing Thompson-sponsored research in 1992. See Morgan and Funderburk, "Phenylpropanolamine and Blood Pressure," 206S–10S.

75 Sack and Mundy, "A Dose of Denial." See also US Food and Drug Administration, Center For Drug Evaluation and Research, Nonprescription Drug Advisory Committee (NDAC) Hearings, *Meeting on Safety Issues of Phenylpropanolamine (PPA) in Over-the-Counter Drug Products*, 19 October 2000, 37–8.

76 FDA, NDAC Hearings, 2000, 39.

77 Gerth and Stolberg, "Another Part of the Battle," 8, and US Food and Drug Administration, Center for Drug Evaluation and Research, *Epidemiologic Review of of Phenylpropanolamine Safety Issues*, 30 April 1991, 1–34.

78 FDA, NDAC Hearings, 2000, 39.

79 Gerth and Stolberg, "Another Part of the Battle," 8.

80 Ibid.

81 Federal Register, Department of Health and Human Services, *Phenylpropanolamine-Containing Drug Products for Over-the-Counter Human Use; Tentative Final Monographs*, 22 December 2005, 70.

82 Ibid.

83 Kernan et al., "Phenylpropanolamine," 1832.

84 Gerth and Stolberg, "Another Part of the Battle," 8.

85 Federal Register, *Phenylpropanolamine-Containing Drug Products for Over-the-Counter Human Use; Tentative Final Monographs*, 2005.

86 Sack and Mundy, "A Dose of Denial."

87 FDA, NDAC Hearings, 2000, 123.

88 Ibid., 111.

89 Ibid., 101.

90 Ibid., 124–5.

91 Ibid.

92 Ibid.

93 Ibid., 164–5.

94 Ibid.

95 Ibid., 173.

96 Ibid., 27.

97 Ibid., 28.

98 Ibid., 27–8.

99 Federal Register, *Phenylpropanolamine-Containing Drug Products for Over-the-Counter Human Use; Tentative Final Monographs*, 2005.

100 Ibid.

101 Ibid.

102 Christine Bittar, "Warnings Against PPA Spell No Relief," *Brandweek* 42, no. 23 (June 2001): S64.

103 US Food and Drug Administration, Department of Health and Human Services, "FDA Letter to Manufacturers of Drug Products Containing Phenylpropanolamine (PPA)," 3 November 2000, http://www.fda.gov/Drugs/DrugSafety/InformationbyDrugClass/ucm150774.htm.

104 Sack and Mundy, "A Dose of Denial."

105 Ibid.

106 Ibid.

107 Kleinfield, "The Ever-Fatter Business of Thinness."

108 Ibid.

109 Ibid.

110 Andrew Pollack, "Side Effects of Diet Pill Still Concern Regulators," *New York Times*, 17 February 2012.

111 Lauren Cooper, "Weight Loss Supplements Found to Contain a Dangerous Drug," *Consumer Reports*, 7 April 2016, http://www.consumerreports.org/health/weight-loss-supplements-found-to-contain-a-dangerous-drug-/.

112 Yen and Ewald, "Toxicity of Weight Loss Agents," 142–52.

CHAPTER EIGHT

1 National Library of Medicine, "Ketamine," *Toxnet: Toxicology Data Network*, accessed 18 October 2016, https://toxnet.nlm.nih.gov/cgi-bin/sis/search/a?dbs+hsdb:@term+@DOCNO+2180; U.S. Food and Drug Administration, "Regulatory Information," accessed 18 October 2016, http://www.fda.gov/Regulatory Information/Legislation/ucm148726.htm.

2 Andrew Pollack, "Special K, a Hallucinogen, Raises Hopes and Concerns as a Treatment for Depression," *New York Times*, 9 December 2014, http://www.nytimes.com/2014/12/10/business/special-k-a-hallucinogen-raises-hopes-and-concerns-as-a-treatment-for-depression.html? r=1.

3 Thomas Insel, "Director's Blog: Ketamine," *National Institute of Mental Health*, 1 October 2014, http://www.nimh.nih.gov/about/director/2014/ketamine.shtml; Simone Grimm and Milan Scheidegger, "Is Ketamine the Next Big Depression Drug?" *Scientific American*, 1 May 2013, http://www.scientificamerican.com/article/is-ketamine-next-big-depression-drug/.

4 "Novel Drugs for Depression," *The Economist*, 15 October 2016, http://www.economist.com/news/science-and-technology/21708655-new-generation-drugs-could-change-way-depression-treated-novel-drugs.

5 Alex Ballingall, "Ketamine Seen as Promising New Depression Drug," *Toronto Star*, 26 August 2014, https://www.thestar.com/life/health_wellness/2014/08/26/ketamine_seen_as_promising_new_depression_drug.html.

6 Rasmussen et al., "Serial Infusions of Low-Dose Ketamine," 444–50; Haroon Siddique, "Ketamine May Help Treat Depression, UK Study

Finds," *The Guardian*, 3 April 2014, https://www.theguardian.com/society/2014/apr/03/ketamine-could-help-to-treat-depression; James Gallagher, "Ketamine 'Exciting' Depression Therapy," BBC *News*, 3 April 2014, http://www.bbc.co.uk/news/health-26647738.

7   Kate Lyons, "From Ketamine to Cupboard Therapy: The Future of Mental Health Treatment," *The Guardian*, 29 July 2016, https://www.theguardian.com/world/2016/jul/29/from-ketamine-to-cupboard-therapy-the-future-of-mental-health-treatment.

8   Sessa Interview.

9   Zarate et al., "A Randomized Trial of an N-methyl-D-asparate," 861.

10 Lai et al., "Pilot Dose-Response Trial of I.V. Ketamine," 579–84; Krupitsky et al., "Single Versus Repeated Sessions of Ketamine-Assisted Psychotherapy," 13–19.

11 Grinspoon and Bakalar, *Psychedelic Drugs Reconsidered*; Halpern, "The Use of Hallucinogens in the Treatment of Addiction," 177–89. See also Halpern and Pope, "Hallucinogen Persisting Perception Disorder," 109–19.

12 Schatzberg, "A Word to the Wise about Ketamine," 262–4.

13 Alicia Ault, "US Ketamine Clinics Continue to Mushroom with No Regulation," *Medscape*, 9 October 2017; Wilkinson et al., "A Survey of the Clinical, Off-Label Use of Ketamine," 695–6.

14 Akporehwe et al., "Ketamine," 1466.

15 World Health Organization, "WHO Recommends against International Control of Ketamine."

16 Rachel Wright, "Ketamine: Why Not Everyone Wants a Ban," BBC *News*, 13 March 2015, http://www.bbc.com/news/health-31859184.

17 Dong et al., "Ketamine," 4911–13.

18 See Erika Kinetz, "DEA Opens Shop in China to Help Fight Synthetic Drug Trade," CTV *News*, 6 January 2017, http://www.ctvnews.ca/world/dea-opens-shop-in-china-to-help-fight-synthetic-drug-trade-1.3229836; Bisola Obembe, "Not Just a Party Drug: No Ketamine Means No Surgery in Some Developing Countries," *The Guardian*, 3 March 2016, https://www.theguardian.com/global-development-professionals-network/2016/mar/03/not-just-a-party-drug-no-ketamine-means-no-surgery-in-some-developing-countries.

19 Kellner et al., "Electroconvulsive Therapy Is a Standard Treatment; Ketamine Is Not (Yet)," 796; "End the Ban on Psychoactive Drug Research," *Scientific American*.

20 Limb, "Ketamine Should Be Upgraded from Class C to Class B Drug," 1.

21 U.S. Department of Defense, "DoD News Briefing – Secretary Rumsfeld and Gen. Myers," Transcript, 12 February 2002, http://archive.defense.gov/Transcripts/Transcript.aspx?TranscriptID=2636.

22 Gabriel, "Restricting the Sale of 'Deadly Poisons,'" 42. See also Tomes, "Merchants of Health."

23 Daemmrich, "Invisible Monuments," 3, 15.

24 Britten, "Patients' Demands for Prescriptions in Primary Care," 1084–5.

25 Szasz, Our Right to Drugs, ix. It is not only those on the right of politics that advocate for a freer drugs market. This policy is popular with the left too. See Suzanne Moore, "LSD Has Improved My Life, So Why Should the State Decide Whether I Can Take It or Not," The Guardian, 13 April 2016, https://www.theguardian.com/commentisfree/2016/apr/13/lsd-has-improved-my-life-state-hallucinogenic-drugs-suzanne-moore.

26 Quoted in McAllister, Drug Diplomacy in the Twentieth Century, 9.

27 Blinderman and Billings, "Comfort Care for Patients Dying in the Hospital," 2549–61.

28 Dan Malleck, "Why Is Everyone Talking about Painkillers, but Not about Pain?" Globe and Mail, 5 January 2017, https://www.theglobeandmail.com/opinion/why-is-everyone-talking-about-painkillers-but-not-about-pain/article33513858/; Lunt et al., "Implications for the NHS."

29 Huxley, Brave New World, 191.

BIBLIOGRAPHY

ARCHIVAL SOURCES

Library of Congress. Congressional Research Services, Science Policy
    Research Division. Washington, DC.
Library of Parliament. House of Commons Debates. Canadian
    Parliamentary Historical Resources. Ottawa.
Provincial Archives of Saskatchewan. Regina.
R.D. Laing Collection. Special Collections. University of Glasgow.
    Glasgow, Scotland.
Robert J. Dole Archive and Special Collections. University of Kansas.
    Lawrence, KS.
Walter Lear Health Activist Collection, University of Pennsylvania Rare
    Book and Manuscript Library. Philadelphia, PA.

INTERVIEW

Ben Sessa Interview by author. Bristol, England. 31 October 2017.

GOVERNMENT DOCUMENTS

Benson, James S. "State of the Food and Drug Administration." Speech. 18
    May 1990. http://www.fda.gov/NewsEvents/Speeches/ucm107156.htm.
Cleland, Richard L., Walter C. Gross, Laura D. Koss, Matthew Daynard,
    and Karen M. Muoio. "Weight-Loss Advertising: An Analysis of
    Current Trends." *A Report of the Staff of the Federal Trade
    Commission*, September 2002. Accessed 18 October 2016. http://news.
    findlaw.com/hdocs/docs/ftc/902weightlossadsrpt.pdf.

Congressional Budget Office. "Would Prescription Drug Importation Reduce U.S. Drug Spending?" CBO: *Economic and Budget Issue Brief*, 29 April 2004. https://www.cbo.gov/sites/default/files/108th-congress-2003-2004/reports/04-29-prescriptiondrugs.pdf.

Criminal Intelligence Service Canada. Public Safety Canada. "Counterfeit Pharmaceuticals in Canada." August 2006. Accessed 17 March 2016. http://www.cisc.gc.ca/pharmaceuticals/documents/counterfeit_pharmaceuticals_e.pdf.

"FDA Crackdown on Illegal Products." FDA *Consumer* 38, no. 2 (2004): 36–7.

"FDA Takes Significant Steps to Protect Americans from Dangers of Tobacco through New Regulation." FDA Pressroom, 5 May 2016. http://www.fda.gov/NewsEvents/Newsroom/PressAnnouncements/ucm499234.htm.

Federal Register. Department of Health and Human Services. *Phenylpropanolamine-Containing Drug Products for Over-the-Counter Human Use; Tentative Final Monographs*. 22 December 2005.

Grigg, Bill. "Memo." *Health and Human Services (HHS) News*, 25 February 1982.

Health Canada. "Buying Drugs over the Internet." November 2009. Accessed 17 October 2016. http://publications.gc.ca/collections/collection_2010/sc-hc/H13-7-68-2009-eng.pdf.

– *Consumer Information – Cannabis (Marihuana, marijuana)*. Ottawa: Health Canada, 2016. Accessed 18 January 2017. http://publications.gc.ca/collections/collection_2016/sc-hc/H129-20-2016-eng.pdf.

– *Information for Health Care Professionals: Cannabis (Marihuana, Marijuana) and Cannabinoids*. Ottawa: Health Canada, 2013. Accessed 18 January 2017. http://publications.gc.ca/collections/collection_2016/sc-hc/H129-19-2013-eng.pdf.

Insel, Thomas. "Director's Blog: Ketamine." *National Institute of Mental Health*, 1 October 2014. http://www.nimh.nih.gov/about/director/2014/ketamine.shtml.

Lafrenière, Gérald, and Leah Spicer. *Illicit Drugs in Canada 1980–2001: A Review and Analysis of Enforcement Trends, Prepared for the Special Senate Committee on Illegal Drugs*. Library of Parliament, 26 June 2002. http://www.parl.gc.ca/Content/SEN/Committee/371/ille/library/DrugTrends-e.htm.

Legislative Assembly of Ontario. "Therapeutic Use of Heroin." Hansard Transcripts. Official Records for 18 October 1984. http://www.ontla.

on.ca/web/houseproceedings/house_detail.do?locale=en&Parl=
32&Sess=4&Date=1984-10-18#P419_131663.

Mackay, Robin, and Karin Phillips. *The Legal Regulation of Marijuana in
Canada and Selected Other Countries*. Ottawa: Library of Parliament,
2016. Accessed 18 January 2017. http://publications.gc.ca/collections/
collection_2016/bdp-lop/bp/YM32-2-2016-94-eng.pdf.

Meadows, Michele. "Imported Drugs Raise Safety Concerns." *FDA
Consumer* 36, no. 5 (2002): 18–23.

Scott, John F., and E.M. Sellers. *Cancer Pain, A Monograph on the
Management of Cancer Pain: A Report of the Expert Advisory
Committee on the Management of Severe Chronic Pain in Cancer
Patients*. Ottawa: Health and Welfare Canada, 1984.

Stone, Brad. "How AIDS Has Changed FDA." *FDA Consumer* 24, no. 1
(February 1990).

Task Force on Marijuana Legalization and Regulation. *Toward the
Legalization, Regulation and Restriction of Access to Marijuana:
Discussion Paper*. Ottawa: Government of Canada, 2016. Accessed 18
January 2017. http://publications.gc.ca/collections/collection_2016/jus/
J11-2016-1-eng.pdf.

US Congress. House of Representatives. Committee on Interstate and
Foreign Commerce. *Drug Regulation Reform – Oversight, New
Drug Approval Process: Hearings before the Subcommittee on Health
and the Environment of the House of Representatives*. 96th Congress,
25 June 1980.

– Committee on Government Operations. *FDA's Regulation of Zomax*,
98th Congress, 1st Session. 26 and 27 April 1983.

– Committee on Science and Technology. *Drug Lag*. 97th Congress, 1st
Session. 16 September 1981.

– House Select Committee on Aging. "Diet Pills." 98th Congress, 1st
Session. 1983.

– Subcommittee on Health and the Environment. *Compassionate Pain
Relief Act: Hearings on H.R. 4762*. 98th Congress, 1985.

– Subcommittee on Health and Scientific Research and Committee on
Human Resources. "Testimony of Louis Lasagna, M.D. on Drug
Regulation Reform Act of 1978." Rochester, NY: The Center for the
Study of Drug Development, 12 April 1978.

– Testimony of William K. Hubbard, Associate Commissioner for Policy,
Planning and Legislation. *Canadian Prescription Drug Reimportation:
Is There a Safety Issue?* Hearings Before the Committee on Government
Reform and Wellness. 108th Congress, 12 June 2003.

– Testimony of William K. Hubbard, Associate Commissioner for Policy, Planning and Legislation. Hearing Before the Committee on Commerce, Science and Transportation. 107th Congress, 5 September 2001.

– Testimony of William K. Hubbard, Associate Commissioner for Policy, Planning and Legislation. *The Importation of Drugs into the United States.* Hearings Before the Committee on Energy and Commerce. 107th Congress, 25 July 2002.

US Congress. Senate. *Dietary Goals for the United States.* Prepared by the Staff of the Select Committee on Nutrition and Human Needs. 95th Congress, 1st Session. February 1977.

– Hearings Before the Select Committee on Nutrition and Human Needs. *National Nutrition Policy Study, 1974.* 93rd Congress, 2nd Session. June 1974.

– Senate Republican Policy Committee. *Legislative Notice: S.1082 – The FDA Revitalization Act.* Number 13. 30 April 2007.

– Testimony of William K. Hubbard, Associate Commissioner for Policy, Planning and Legislation. *The Importation of Drugs into the United States.* Hearings Before the Special Committee on Aging. 107th Congress, 9 June 2002.

– Testimony of William K. Hubbard and John M. Taylor. *A System Overwhelmed: The Avalanche of Imported, Counterfeit and Unapproved Drugs in the U.S.* Hearings before the Committee on Governmental Affairs. 108th Congress, 24 June 2003.

US Department of Defense. "DoD News Briefing – Secretary Rumsfeld and Gen. Myers." Transcript. 12 February 2002. http://archive.defense.gov/Transcripts/Transcript.aspx?TranscriptID=2636.

US Department of Health, Education, and Welfare. *Review Panel on New Drug Regulation: Final Report.* Washington, DC: Department of Health, Education, and Welfare, 1977.

US Food and Drug Administration. Center for Drug Evaluation and Research. *Epidemiologic Review of of Phenylpropanolamine Safety Issues.* 30 April 1991.

– Center for Drug Evaluation and Research. Nonprescription Drug Advisory Committee (NDAC) Hearings. *Meeting on Safety Issues of Phenylpropanolamine (PPA) in Over-the Counter Drug Products.* 19 October 2000.

– Department of Health and Human Services. *FDA Counterfeit Drug Task Force Interim Report.* October 2003.

– Department of Health and Human Services. "FDA Letter to Manufacturers of Drug Products Containing Phenylpropanolamine

(PPA)." 3 November 2000. http://www.fda.gov/Drugs/DrugSafety/
InformationbyDrugClass/ucm150774.htm.

– FDA *Quarterly Activities Report*, FY 1978, 1st Quarter. Washington, DC:
1975.

– "Regulatory Information." Accessed 18 October 2016. http://www.fda.
gov/RegulatoryInformation/Legislation/ucm148726.htm.

SECONDARY SOURCES

Aaronson, Bernard, and Humphry Osmond, eds. *Psychedelics: The Uses
and Implications of Hallucinogenic Drugs*. Garden City, NY: Anchor,
1970.

Abraham, John. *Science, Politics and the Pharmaceutical Industry:
Controversy and Bias in Drug Regulation*. New York: St. Martin's
Press, 1995.

Abramson, Harold. *The Use of LSD in Psychotherapy: Transactions of a
Conference on d Lysergic Acid Diethylamide (LSD-25)*. Princeton, NJ:
Josiah Macy Foundation, 1960.

Acker, Carolyn Jean. *Creating the American Junkie: Addiction Research in
the Classic Era of Narcotic Control*. Baltimore, MD: Johns Hopkins
University Press, 2002.

Akporehwe, Nosa A., Paul R. Wilkinson, Rachel Quibell, and Kerstine A.
Akporehwe. "Ketamine: A Misunderstood Analgesic." *BMJ: British
Medical Journal* 332, no. 7556 (2006): 1466.

Angell, Marcia. *The Truth about Drug Companies: How They Deceive Us
and What to Do about It*. New York: Random House, 2004.

Appleson, Gail. "Agencies Probe Safety of Cold, Diet Medicine." *American
Bar Association Journal* 68, no. 12 (1982): 1558.

Avorn, Jerry. *Powerful Medicines: The Benefits, Risks, and Costs of
Prescription Drugs*. New York: Knopf, 2004.

Baer, Hans. *Biomedicine and Alternative Healing Systems in America:
Issues of Class, Race, Ethnicity, and Gender*. Madison: University of
Wisconsin Press, 2001.

Barber, Patrick. *Psychedelic Revolutionaries: LSD Pioneers and the Rise
and Fall of Hallucinogenic Research*. Regina: University of Regina
Press, 2017.

Barron, Stanley, Eugene Ebner, and Paul Lowinger. "A Clinical
Examination of Chronic LSD Use in the Community." *Comprehensive
Psychiatry* 11 (January 1970): 69–79.

Barry, Rachel Ann, et al. "Waiting for the Opportune Moment: The Tobacco Industry and Marijuana Legalization." *The Milbank Quarterly* 92, no. 2 (2014): 207–42.

Batchelor, Bob, and Scott Stoddart. *The 1980s*. Westport, CT: Greenwood Press, 2007.

Bennet, Glin. "LSD: 1967." *The British Journal of Psychiatry* 114 (1968): 1219–22.

Benshoff, Harry M. "The Short-Lived Life of the Hollywood LSD Film." *Velvet Light Trap* 47 (2001): 29–44.

Berry, I., and R. Martin, eds. *The Pharmaceutical Regulatory Process*. New York: Informa Healthcare, 2008.

Bhosle, Monali J., and Rajesh Balkrishnan. "Drug Reimportation Practices in the United States." *Therapeutics and Clinical Risk Management* 3, no. 1 (2007): 41–6.

Blinderman, Craig D., and J. Andrew Billings. "Comfort Care for Patients Dying in the Hospital." *New England Journal of Medicine* 373 (2015): 2549–61.

Bloom, Sandra. *Creating Sanctuary: Toward the Evolution of Sane Societies*. New York: Routledge, 2013.

Boerner, Udo, Seth Abbott, and Robert L. Roe. "The Metabolism of Morphine and Heroin in Man." *Drug Metabolism Review* 4, no. 1 (1975): 39–73.

Bourke, Joanna. *The Story of Pain: From Prayers to Painkillers*. Oxford, UK: Oxford University Press, 2014.

Boyd, Susan. *From Witches to Crack Moms: Women, Drugs Laws, and Policy*. Durham, NC: Carolina Academic Press, 2004.

Bradford, Robert W., and Michael L. Culbert. "The Laetrile Phenomenon – Harbinger of Medical Revolution." *Jurimetrics Journal* 21, no. 2 (1980): 179–93.

Brandt, Allan M. *The Cigarette Century: The Rise, Fall, and Deadly Persistence of the Product that Defined America*. New York: Basic Books, 2009.

Brecher, Edward M. *Licit and Illicit Drugs: The Consumers Union Report on Narcotics, Stimulants, Depressants, Inhalants, Hallucinogens, and Marijuana – Including Caffeine, Nicotine, and Alcohol*. Boston, MA: Little, Brown & Company, 1972.

Breyer, Stephen. *Breaking the Vicious Circle: Toward Effective Risk Regulation*. Cambridge, MA: Harvard University Press, 1993.

Britten, Nicky. "Patients' Demands for Prescriptions in Primary Care: Patients Cannot Take All the Blame for Overprescribing." *BMJ: British Medical Journal* 310, no. 6977 (1995): 1084–5.

Brown, Walter A. "Research on Psychedelics Making a Comeback." *Applied Neurology* 3 (2007): 23–7.

Buckingham, Robert W. "Hospice and Health Policy." *Health Policy and Education* 1, no. 4 (1980): 303–15.

Burkholz, Herbert. *The FDA Follies*. New York: Basic Books, 1994.

Burroughs, William. *Junkie*. New York: Penguin Books, 1987.

Burston, Daniel. *The Crucible of Experience: R.D. Laing and the Crisis of Psychotherapy*. Cambridge: Harvard University Press, 2000.

Callahan, Daniel, and Sissela Bok, eds. *Ethics Teaching in Higher Education*. New York: Plenum Press, 1980.

Campbell, Lara, Dominique Clément, and Gregory S. Kealey, eds. *Debating Dissent: Canada and the Sixties*. Toronto: University of Toronto Press, 2012.

Campos, Alline Cristina, et al. "Multiple Mechanisms Involved in the Large-Spectrum Therapeutic Potential of Cannabidiol in Psychiatric Disorders." *Philosophical Transactions: Biological Sciences* 367, no. 1607 (2012): 3364–78.

Canadian Medical Association. "CMA Policy: CMA Statement, Authorizing Marijuana for Medical Purposes (Update 2015)." http://policybase.cma. ca/dbtw-wpd/Policypdf/PD15-04.pdf (accessed 14 October 2016).

Caplan, Gerald. *Principles of Preventive Psychiatry*. New York: Basic Books, 1964.

Carnwath, Tom, and Ian White. *Heroin Century*. New York: Routledge, 2002.

Carpenter, Daniel. *Reputation and Power: Organizational Image and Pharmaceutical Regulation at the FDA*. Princeton, NJ: Princeton University Press, 2010.

Cayleff, Susan E. *Nature's Path: A History of Naturopathic Healing in America*. Baltimore, MD: JHUP, 2016.

Centre for Addiction and Mental Health. "Cannabis Policy Framework." October 2014. https://www.camh.ca/en/hospital/about_camh/ influencing_public_policy/documents/camhcannabispolicyframework. pdf (accessed 31 January 2017).

Chasin, Alexandra. *Assassin of Youth: A Kaleidoscopic History of Harry J. Anslinger's War on Drugs*. Chicago, IL: University of Chicago Press, 2016.

Clark, David. *To Comfort Always: A History of Palliative Care since the 19th Century*. Oxford, UK: Oxford University Press, 2016.

Clow, Barbara. "Mahlon William Locke: 'Toe-Twister.'" *Canadian Bulletin of Medical History* 9 (1992): 17–39.

Cohen, I. Glenn. *Patients with Passports: Medical Tourism, Law, and Ethics*. New York: Oxford University Press, 2014.

Cohen, I. Glenn, and Holly Fernandez Lynch, eds. FDA *in the 21st Century: The Challenges of Regulating Drugs and New Technologies*. New York: Columbia University Press, 2015.

Cohen, I. Glenn, Holly Fernandez Lynch, and Christopher T. Robertson, eds. *Nudging Health: Health Law and Behavioral Economics*. Baltimore, MD: Johns Hopkins University Press, 2016.

Cohen, Jillian Clare. "Public Policy Implications of Cross-Border Internet Pharmacies." *Managed Care* 13, no. 3 (2004): 14–16.

– "Pushing the Borders: The Moral Dilemma of International Internet Pharmacies." *Hastings Center Report* 34, no. 2 (2004): 15–17.

Cohen, Marcus A. "Michael L. Culbert, ScD, Fighter for Health Freedom (1937–2004)." *Townsend Letter for Doctors & Patients* 258 (2005): 16–17.

Cohen, Steven P. "Cannabinoids for Chronic Pain." BMJ: *British Medical Journal* 336, no. 7637 (2008): 167–8.

College of Family Physicians of Canada, the. "The College of Family Physicians of Canada Statement on Health Canada's Proposed Changes to Medical Marijuana Regulations." February 2013. http://www.cfpc.ca/uploadedFiles/Health_Policy/CFPC_Policy_Papers_and_Endorsements/CFPC_Policy_Papers/Medical%20Marijuana%20Position%20Statement%20CFPC.pdf (accessed 14 October 2016).

College of Physicians and Surgeons of British Columbia. "Professional Standards and Guidelines: Marijuana for Medical Purposes." 30 July 2015. https://www.cpsbc.ca/files/pdf/PSG-Marijuana-for-Medical-Purposes.pdf (accessed 14 October 2016).

College of Physicians and Surgeons of Saskatchewan. "Prescribing Medical Marihuana." June 2014. http://www.cps.sk.ca/imis/Documents/Brochures/Marihuana Regulations_mailout-web.pdf (accessed 14 October 2016).

Collins, Harry, and Trevor Pinch. *Dr. Golem: How to Think about Medicine*. Chicago, IL: University of Chicago Press, 2005.

Collins, Robert M. *Transforming America: Politics and Culture in the Reagan Years*. New York: Columbia University Press, 2008.

Comeau, Pauline, Heather Kent, Lisa Gregoire, and Barbara Sibbald. "News @ a Glance." *Canadian Medical Association Journal* 171, no. 11 (2004): 1336.

Committee on the Health Effects of Marijuana: An Evidence Review and Research Agenda. *The Health Effects of Cannabis and Cannabinoids: The Current State of Evidence and Recommendations for Research.* Washington, DC: The National Academies Press, 2017.

"Congress Considers Safety of Diet Aids." *American Pharmacy* 23, no. 9 (1983): 448.

Cornwell, Benjamin, and Annulla Linders. "'The Myth of 'Moral Panic': An Alternative Account of LSD Prohibition." *Deviant Behavior* 23, no. 4 (2002): 307–30.

Courtwright, David. *Dark Paradise: Opiate Addiction in America before 1940.* Cambridge: Harvard University Press, 1982.

Crippen, David W., and Robert M. Veatch. "Laetrile: Cancer Cure or Quack Remedy?" *Hastings Center Report* 6, no. 6 (1976): 18–20.

Culbert, Michael L. *Freedom from Cancer: The Amazing Story of Vitamin B-17, or Laetrile.* Seal Beach, CA: '76 Press, 1976.

– *Vitamin B-17 – Forbidden Weapon Against Cancer: The Fight for Laetrile.* New Rochelle, NY: Arlington House, 1974.

Daemmrich, Arthur. "Invisible Monuments and the Costs of Pharmaceutical Regulation: Twenty-Five Years of Drug Lag Debate." *Pharmacy in History* 45, no. 1 (2003): 3–17.

– *Pharmacopolitics: Drug Regulation in the United States and Germany.* Chapel Hill, NC: University of North Carolina Press, 2004.

Daemmrich, Arthur, and Joanna Radin, eds. *Perspectives on Risk and Regulation: The FDA at 100.* Philadelphia: Chemical Heritage Foundation, 2007.

Daratsos, Louisa, and Judith L. Howe. "The Development of Palliative Care Programs in the Veterans Administration: Zelda Foster's Legacy." *Journal of Social Work in End-of-Life & Palliative Care* 3, no. 1 (2007): 29–39.

Da Sylva, Normand P. "The CMA's Stand on the Medical Use of Heroin: Setting the Record Straight." *Canadian Medical Association Journal* 130, no. 12 (1984): 1515.

De Spain, June. *The Little Cyanide Cookbook: Delicious Recipes Rich in Vitamin B-17.* Thousand Oaks, CA: American Media, 1976.

Dickin, Janice. "'Take Up Thy Bed and Walk': Aimee Semple McPherson and Faith-Healing." *Canadian Bulletin of Medical History* 17, no. 1 (2000): 137–53.

Dickinson, Harley. *The Two Psychiatries: The Transformation of Psychiatric Work in Saskatchewan, 1905–1984.* Regina: Canadian Plains Research Centre, 1989.

Dickinson, James G. "Gingrich Plan for the FDA Leaves Questions." *Medical Marketing and Media* 31 (March 1995): 10.

Dittmer, John. *The Good Doctors: The Medical Committee for Human Rights and the Struggle for Social Justice in Health Care.* New York: Bloomsbury Press, 2009.

Dixon, Bernard. "Schizophrenia Controversy." *British Medical Journal* 298, no. 6668 (1989): 265.

Dodgson, Rick. *It's All a Kind of Magic: The Young Ken Kesey.* Madison: University of Wisconsin Press, 2013.

Dong, T.T., J. Mellin-Olsen, and A.W. Gelb. "Ketamine: A Growing Global Health-Care Need." *British Journal of Anaesthesia* 115, no. 4 (2015): 4911–13.

Drake, Nadia. "Forty Years On from Nixon's War, Cancer Research 'Evolves.'" *Nature Medicine* 17, no. 7 (2011): 757.

Dreyfuss, Robert. "Popping Contributions: The New Battle for the FDA." *The American Prospect* 33 (July/August 1997): 53–9.

Duffin, Jacalyn. "Palliative Care: The Oldest Profession?" *Canadian Bulletin for the History of Medicine* 31, no. 2 (2014): 205–28.

Dyck, Erika. "Hitting Highs at Rock Bottom: LSD Treatment for Alcoholism, 1950–1970." *Social History of Medicine* 19, no. 2 (2006): 313–30.

– "Land of the Living Skies with Diamonds: A Place for Radical Psychiatry?" *Journal of Canadian Studies* 41, no. 3 (2007): 42–66.

– *Psychedelic Psychiatry: LSD from Clinic to Campus.* Baltimore, MD: Johns Hopkins University Press, 2008.

Dyck, Erika, and Tolly Bradford. "Peyote on the Prairies: Religion, Scientists and Native Newcomer Relations in Western Canada." *Journal of Canadian Studies* 46, no. 1 (2012): 28–52.

Eggerston, Laura. "Health Minister Ends Special Access to Prescription Heroin." *Canadian Medical Association Journal* 185, no. 17 (2013): E773–4.

Eliot, Marc. *Steve McQueen.* New York: Three Rivers Press, 2011.

Ellwood, Robert S. *The Sixties Spiritual Awakening: American Religion Moving from Modern to Postmodern.* New Brunswick, NJ: Rutgers University Press, 1994.

Emerson, Amy, et al. "History and Future of the Multidisciplinary Association for Psychedelic Studies (MAPS)." *Journal of Psychoactive Drugs* 46, no. 1 (2014): 27–36.

Engel, Jonathan. *The Epidemic: A Global History of AIDS.* New York: Smithsonian Books, 2006.

Farber, David, and Beth Bailey, eds. *America in the 1970s.* Lawrence, KS: University Press of Kansas, 2000.

"FDA in 1996: Twice as NCE." *Medical Marketing and Media* 32 (27 February 1996).

Finkelstein, Eric A., and Laurie Zuckerman. *The Fattening of America: How the Economy Makes Us Fat, If It Matters, and What to Do about It.* New York: Wiley, 2007.

Finkelstein, Stan, and Peter Temin. *Reasonable RX: Solving the Drug Price Crisis.* Upper Saddle River, NJ: FT Press, 2008.

Fischer, Benedikt, Sharan Kuganesan, and Robin Room. "Medical Marijuana Programs: Implications for Cannabis Control Policy – Observations from Canada." *International Journal of Drug Policy* 26, no. 1 (2015): 15–19.

Fischer, Benedikt, Jürgen Rehm, and Jean-François Crépault. "Realistically Furthering the Goals of Public Health by Cannabis Legalization with Strict Regulation: Response to Kalant." *International Journal of Drug Policy* 34 (2016): 11–16.

Fischer, Benedikt, Jürgen Rehm, and Wayne Hall. "Cannabis Use in Canada: The Need for a 'Public Health' Approach." *Canadian Journal of Public Health* 100, no. 2 (2009): 101–3.

Foley, Kathleen F. "Controversies in Cancer Pain: Medical Perspectives." *Cancer* 63, no. 11 (1989): 2257–65.

Foreman, Judy. *A Nation in Pain: Healing Our Biggest Health Problem.* Oxford, UK: Oxford University Press, 2014.

Foster, Zelda. "How Social Work Can Influence Hospital Management of Fatal Illness." *Social Work* 10, no. 4 (1965): 30–5.

Fuchs, Edward P., and James Anderson. "The Institutionalization of Cost-Benefit Analysis." *Public Productivity Review* 10, no. 4 (1987): 25–33.

Fukuyama, Francis. *Our Posthuman Future: Consequences of the Biotechnology Revolution.* London: Profile Books, 2003.

Furst, Peter T. *Flesh of the Gods: The Ritual Use of Hallucinogens.* London: Wavelength Press, 1990.

Furth, Charlotte. "The AMS/Paterson Lecture: Becoming Alternative? Modern Transformations of Chinese Medicine in China and in the

United States." *Canadian Bulletin of Medical History* 28, no. 1 (2011): 5–41.

Gabriel, Joseph M. "Restricting the Sale of 'Deadly Poisons': Pharmacists, Drug Regulation, and Narratives of Suffering in the Gilded Age." *Pharmacy in History* 53, no. 1 (2011): 29–45.

– *Medical Monopoly: Intellectual Property Rights and the Origins of the Modern Pharmaceutical Industry.* Chicago, IL: University of Chicago Press, 2014.

Gallagher, Mark. "Tripped Out: The Psychedelic Film and Masculinity." *Quarterly Review of Film and Video* 21, no. 3 (2004): 161–71.

Gapstur, Susan M., and Michael J. Thun. "Progress in the War on Cancer." *Journal of the American Medical Association* 303, no. 11 (2010): 1084–5.

Gardner, Martha M., and Allan Brandt. "'The Doctors' Choice Is America's Choice': The Physician in US Cigarette Advertisements, 1930–1953." *American Journal of Public Health* 96, no. 2 (2006): 222–32.

Ghent, W.R. "Heroin – Panacea or Plague." *Queen's Quarterly* 93, no. 4 (1986): 808–20.

Giacomini, Kathleen M., et al. "When Good Drugs Go Bad." *Nature* 446, no. 7139 (2007): 975–7.

Gibson, A.C. "How ECT Works." *British Medical Journal* 4, no. 5989 (1975): 169.

Gifford-Jones, W. *You're Going to Do What?: The Memoir of Dr. W. Gifford-Jones.* Toronto: ECW Press, 2000.

Gill, Oliver. "Hospice Pioneer." *Nursing Standard* 13, no. 47 (1999): 18.

Glasser, Barry. "Fitness and the Postmodern Self." *Journal of Health and Social Behavior* 30, no. 2 (1989): 180–91.

Goode, Erich, and Ben-Yehuda Nachman. *Moral Panics: The Social Construction of Deviance.* Oxford, UK: Wiley-Blackwell, 2009.

Gorman, Dennis M. "'War on Drugs' Continues in United States Under New Leadership." *British Medical Journal Clinical Research* 307, no. 6900 (1993): 369–71.

Graham, John R., ed. *What States Can Do to Reform Health Care: A Free-Market Primer.* San Francisco, CA: Pacific Research Institute, 2006.

Greene, Jeremy. *Generic: The Unbranding of Modern Medicine.* Baltimore, MD: John Hopkins University Press, 2014.

Greene, Jeremy A. *Prescribing by Numbers: Drugs and the Definition of Disease.* Baltimore, MD: Johns Hopkins University Press, 2007.

Greene, Jeremy, and David Herzberg. "Hidden in Plain Sight: Marketing Prescription Drugs to Consumers in the Twentieth Century." *American Journal of Public Health* 100, no. 5 (May 2010): 793–803.

Greenfield, Robert. *Timothy Leary: A Biography.* Orlando, FL: Harcourt, Inc., 2006.

Griffin, Edward G. *World without Cancer: The Story of Vitamin B-17.* Thousand Oaks, CA: American Media, 1974.

Grinspoon, Lester, and J. Bakalar. *Psychedelic Drugs Reconsidered.* New York: Basic Books, 1979.

Grof, Stanislav. *Realms of the Human Unconscious: Observations from LSD Research.* New York: Viking Press, 1975.

Grossman, Lewis A. "The Rise of the Empowered Consumer." *Regulation* 37, no. 4 (Winter 2014–15): 34–41.

Gundle, Kenneth R., et al. "'To Prove This Is the Industry's Best Hope': Big Tobacco's Support of Research on the Genetics of Nicotine Addiction." *Addiction* 105, no. 6 (2010): 974–83.

Halberstam, David. *War in a Time of Peace: Bush, Clinton, and the Generals.* New York: Scribner, 2001.

Halpern, John H. "The Use of Hallucinogens in the Treatment of Addiction." *Addiction Research* 4, no. 2 (1996): 177–89.

Halpern, John H., and Harrison Pope Jr. "Hallucinogen Persisting Perception Disorder: What Do We Know after 50 Years?" *Drug and Alcohol Dependence* 69, no. 2 (2003): 109–19.

Hari, Johann. *Chasing the Scream: The First and Last Days of the War on Drugs.* London: Bloomsbury, 2015.

Harris, Louis S., ed. *Problems of Drug Dependence 1996: Proceedings of the 58th Annual Scientific Meeting, The College on Problems of Drug Dependence Inc.* Rockville, MD: National Institute on Drug Abuse, 1997.

Hawthorne, Fran. *Inside the FDA: The Business and Politics Behind the Drugs We Take and the Food We Eat.* Hoboken, NJ: Wiley, 2005.

Healy, David. *The Creation of Psychopharmacology.* Cambridge: Harvard University Press, 2002.

– *Let Them Eat Prozac: The Unhealthy Relationship between the Pharmaceutical Industry and Depression.* New York: New York University Press, 2004.

– *Mania: A Short History of Bipolar Disorder.* Baltimore, MD: Johns Hopkins University Press, 2008.

Henry, John A., et al. "Comparing Cannabis With Tobacco: Smoking
    Cannabis, Like Smoking Tobacco, Can Be a Public Health Hazard."
    BMJ: British Medical Journal 336, no. 7396 (2003): 942–3.

"Heroin for Cancer: A Great Non-issue of Our Day." *The Lancet* 323, no.
    8392 (June 30, 1984): 1449–50.

Herzberg, David. *Happy Pills in America: From Miltown to Prozac.*
    Baltimore, MD: Johns Hopkins University Press, 2009.

– "Entitled to Addiction? Pharmaceuticals, Race, and America's First Drug
    War." *Bulletin of the History of Medicine* 91, no. 3 (Fall 2017):
    586–623.

Hickman, Meredith A., ed. *The Food and Drug Administration.* New
    York: Nova Science Publishers, 2003.

Hickman, Timothy. "Drugs and Race in American Culture: Orientalism in
    the Turn of the Century Discourse of Narcotic Addiction." *American
    Studies* 41, no. 1 (2000): 71–91.

Hill, Matthew. "Perspective: Be Clear about the Real Risks." *Nature* 525,
    no. 7570 (2015): S14.

Hilts, Philip J. *Protecting America's Health: The FDA, Business, and One
    Hundred Years of Regulation.* New York: Knopf, 2003.

Hodges, Jill R., Ann Marie Kimball, and Leigh Turner, eds. *Risks and
    Challenges in Medical Tourism: Understanding the Global Market for
    Health Services.* New York: Praeger, 2012.

Hoffer, Abram, and Humphry Osmond. *The Hallucinogens.* New York:
    Academic Press, 1967.

Hofmann, Albert. *LSD: My Problem Child and Insights/Outlooks.* Oxford,
    UK: Oxford University Press, 2013.

Holden, Constance. "Drug Abuse 1975: The 'War' Is Past, the Problem Is
    Big as Ever." *Science* 190, no. 4215 (1975): 638–41.

– "Laetrile: 'Quack' Cancer Remedy Still Brings Hope to Sufferers."
    Science 194, no. 4257 (1976): 982–5.

Hollingshead, August. "Some Issues in the Epidemiology of
    Schizophrenia." *American Sociological Review* 26, no. 1 (1961): 5–13.

Horgan, John. "The Electric Kool-Aid Clinical Trial: LSD and Other
    Hallucinogens Were Once Considered Promising Psychiatric
    Treatments." *New Scientist* 185, no. 2488 (2005): 36–40.

Horwitz, Robert B. "Understanding Deregulation." *Theory and Society* 15
    (1986): 139–74.

Huxley, Aldous. *Brave New World.* Toronto: Indigo Library, 2015.

Hynes, William J., and William G. Doty, eds. *Mythical Trickster Figures: Contours, Contexts and Criticisms*. Tuscaloosa, AL, and London: University of Alabama Press, 1993.

Iversen, Les. "Comparing Cannabis with Tobacco: Arithmetic Does Not Add Up." *BMJ: British Medical Journal* 327, no. 7407 (2003): 165.

Jackson, Donald Dale. "The Art of Wishful Shrinking Has Made a Lot of People Rich." *Smithsonian Magazine* 25, no. 8 (1994): 146–56.

Jackson, Kathy Merlock, Lisa Lyon Payne, and Kathy Shepherd Stolley. *The Intersection of Star Culture in America and International Medical Tourism: Celebrity Treatment*. Lanham, MD: Lexington Books, 2016.

Jenkins, Philip. *Decade of Nightmares: The End of the Sixties and the Making of Eighties America*. New York: Oxford University Press, 2006.

Jonnes, Jill. *Hep-Cats, Narcs, and Pipe Dreams: A History of America's Romance with Illegal Drugs*. Baltimore, MD: Johns Hopkins University Press, 1996.

Kagan, Elizabeth, and Margaret Morse. "The Body Electronic: Aerobic Exercise on Video: Women's Search for Empowerment and Self-Transformation." *TDR* 32, no. 4 (1988): 164–80.

Kahan, Meldon, et al. "Prescribing Smoked Cannabis for Chronic Noncancer Pain." *Canadian Family Physician* 60, no. 12 (2014): 1083–90.

Kaiko, Robert F., et al. "Analgesic and Mood Effects of Heroin and Morphine in Cancer Patients with Postoperative Pain." *New England Journal of Medicine* 304, no. 25 (1981): 1501–5.

Kaiser, David, and Patrick McCray, eds. *Groovy Science: Knowledge, Innovation, and American Counterculture*. Chicago, IL: University of Chicago Press, 2016.

Kalant, Harold. "Cannabis Control Policy: No Rational Basis Yet for Legalization." *Clinical Pharmacology & Therapeutics* 97, no. 6 (2015): 538–40.

– "A Critique of Cannabis Legalization Proposals in Canada." *International Journal of Drug Policy* 34 (2016): 5–10.

Kalman, Laura. *Right Star Rising: A New Politics, 1974–1980*. New York: W.W. Norton & Company, 2010.

Kamienski, Lukasz. *Shooting Up: A Short History of Drugs and War*. New York: Oxford University Press, 2016.

Kaplan, John. *The Hardest Drug: Heroin and Public Policy*. Chicago, IL: University of Chicago Press, 1983.

Kellner, Charles H., Robert M. Greenberg, Gabriella M. Ahle, and Lauren S. Liebman. "Electroconvulsive Therapy Is a Standard Treatment; Ketamine Is Not (Yet)." *American Journal of Psychiatry* 171, no. 7 (2014): 796.

Kelly, J.P. "Fractures Complicate ECT." *British Medical Journal* 2, no. 4879 (1954): 98–9.

Kernan, Walter N., Catherine Viscoli, Lawrence Brass, Joseph Broderick, Thomas Brott, Edward Feldmann, Lewis B. Morgenstein, Janet Lee Wilterdink, and Ralph I. Horwitz. "Phenylpropanolamine and the Risk of Hemorrhagic Stroke." *New England Journal of Medicine* 343, no. 25 (2000): 1826–32.

Kesey, Ken. *One Flew Over the Cuckoo's Nest.* New York: Viking Press, 1962.

Killen, Andreas. *1973 Nervous Breakdown: Watergate, Warhol and the Birth of Post-Sixties America.* New York: Bloomsbury USA, 2006.

Kittler, Glenn D. *Laetrile (The Anti-Cancer Drug): Control for Cancer.* New York: Paperback Library, 1963.

Krebs, Teri S., and Pål-Ørjan Johansen. "Lysergic Acid Diethylamide (LSD) for Alcoholism: A Meta-analysis of Randomized Controlled Trials." *Journal of Psychopharmacology* 26, no. 7 (2012): 994–1002.

Kripal, Jeffrey J. *Esalen: America and the Religion of No Religion.* Chicago, IL: The University of Chicago Press, 2007.

Krupitsky, Evgeny M., Andrei Burakov, Igor V. Dunaevsky, et al. "Single versus Repeated Sessions of Ketamine-Assisted Psychotherapy for People with Heroin Dependence." *Journal of Psychoactive Drugs* 39, no. 1 (2007): 13–19.

Kuhn, Cynthia, Scott Schwarzwelder, Wilkie Wilson, Leigh Heather Wilson, and Jeremy Foster. *Buzzed: The Straight Facts About the Most Used and Abused Drugs from Alcohol to Ecstasy.* New York: W.W. Norton & Company, 1998.

Kushner, Howard I. "The Other War on Drugs: The Pharmaceutical Industry, Evidence-Based Medicine and Clinical Research." *Journal of Policy History* 19, no. 1 (2007): 49–70.

Kuzmarov, Jeremy. "From Counter-Insurgency to Narco-Insurgency: Vietnam and the International War on Drugs." *The Journal of Policy History* 20, no. 3 (2008): 344–78.

– *The Myth of the Addicted Army: Vietnam and the Modern War on Drugs.* Boston, MA: University of Massachusetts Press, 2009.

Labate, Beatriz Caiuby, and Kevin Feeney. "Ayahuasca and the Process of Regulation in Brazil and Internationally: Implications and Challenges." *International Journal of Drug Policy* 23, no. 2 (2012): 154–61.

Lai, Rosalyn, Natalie Katalinic, Paul Glue, et al. "Pilot Dose-Response Trial of I.V. Ketamine in Treatment-Resistant Depression." *The World Journal of Biological Psychiatry* 15, no. 7 (2014): 579–84.

Lake, C. Raymond, David Rosenberg, and Rose Quirk. "Phenylpropanolamine and Caffeine Use among Diet Center Clients." *International Journal of Obesity* 14, no. 7 (1990): 575–82.

Lake, Stephanie, Thomas Kerr, and Julio Montaner. "Prescribing Medical Cannabis in Canada: Are We Being Too Cautious?" *Canadian Journal of Public Health* 106, no. 5 (2015): E328–30. *The Lancet Psychiatry* 4, no. 5 (May 2017): 347–426.

Landau, Emanuel. "Review of *World Without Cancer: The Story of Vitamin B-17*, by G. Edward Griffin." *American Journal of Public Health* 66, no. 7 (1976): 696.

Langlitz, Nicolas. *Neuropsychedelia: The Revival of Hallucinogen Research since the Decade of the Brain*. Berkeley, CA: University of California Press, 2013.

Lasagna, Louis. "Heroin: A Medical Me-Too." *New England Journal of Medicine* 304, no. 25 (1981): 1539–40.

– *Phenylpropanolomine – A Review*. New York: John Wiley & Sons, 1988.

Lasek, William, and Steven J.C. Gaulin. "Waist-Hip Ratio and Cognitive Ability: Is Gluteofemoral Fat a Privileged Store of Neurodevelopmental Resources?" *Evolution and Human Behavior* 29, no. 1 (January 2008): 26–34.

Lawler, Andrew, and Richard Stone. "FDA: Congress Mixes Harsh Medicine." *Science* 269 (25 August 1995): 1038–41.

Lee, Martin A. *Smoke Signals: A Social History of Marijuana – Medical, Recreational and Scientific*. New York: Scribner, 2013.

Lenton, Simon. "New Regulated Markets for Recreational Cannabis: Public Health or Private Profit." *Addiction* 109, no. 3 (2014): 354–5.

Lerner, Barron. *When Illness Goes Public: Celebrity Patients and How We Look at Medicine*. Baltimore, MD: Johns Hopkins University Press, 2006.

Lewis, B.J., and V.T. DiVita Jr. "Is There a Place for Heroin in the Symptomatic Support of Cancer Patients?" Unpublished paper. Bethesda, MD: National Cancer Institute, 1977.

Li, Hao, and Wendy Cui. "Patients without Borders: The Historical
    Changes of Medical Tourism." *University of Western Ontario Medical
    Journal* 83, no. 2 (2014): 20–2.
Li, Jie Jack. *Blockbuster Drugs: The Rise and Fall of the Pharmaceutical
    Industry*. New York: Oxford University Press, 2014.
Limb, Matthew. "Ketamine Should Be Upgraded from Class C to Class B
    Drug, Committee Says." BMJ: *British Medical Journal* 347, no. 7937
    (2013): 1.
Loizeau, Pierre-Marie. *Nancy Reagan in Perspective*. New York: Nova
    History Publications, 2005.
– *Nancy Reagan: The Woman Behind the Man*. New York: Nova Science
    Publishers, 2011.
Lough, Shannon. "Growing the Evidence Base for Medical Cannabis."
    Canadian Medical Association Journal 187, no. 13 (2015): 955–6.
Lowe, Mary Frances. "Pharmaceutical Regulatory Policy: A Departmental
    and Administrative Perspective." *Food Drug Cosmetic Law Journal* 39
    (1984): 504–9.
Lowinger, Paul, and Philip Lee Polakoff. "Do Medical Students 'Turn
    On'?" *Comprehensive Psychiatry* 13, no. 2 (1972): 185–8.
Lunde, Anders Steen. "Health in the United States." *Annals of the
    American Academy of Political and Social Science* 453 (1981): 28–69.
Lunt, Neil, and Richard D. Smith, Russell Mannion, Stephen T. Green,
    Mark Exworthy, Johanna Hanefeld, Daniel Horsfall, Laura Machin,
    and Hannah King. "Implications for the NHS of Inward and Outward
    Medical Tourism: A Policy and Economic Analysis Using Literature
    Review and Mixed-Methods Approaches." *Health Services and Delivery
    Research* 2, no. 2 (2015).
Lybecker, Kristen. "Economics of Reimportation and Risks of Counterfeit
    Pharmaceuticals." *Managed Care* 13, no. 3 (2004): 10–14.
Lynch, Mary, and Fiona Campbell. "Cannabinoids for Treatment of
    Chronic Non-cancer pain; A Systematic Review of Randomized Trials."
    British Journal of Clinical Pharmacology 72, no. 5 (2011): 735–44.
Macleod, John, and Matthew Hickman. "How Ideology Shapes the
    Evidence and the Policy: What Do We Know about Cannabis Use and
    What Should We Do?" *Addiction* 105, no. 8 (2010): 1326–30.
– "Response to Commentaries: Moving towards an Evidence-Based Policy
    around Cannabis Use." *Addiction* 105, no. 8 (2010): 1337–9.
Malleck, Dan. *Try to Control Yourself: The Regulation of Public Drinking
    in Post-Prohibition Ontario, 1927–1944*. Vancouver, BC: University of
    British Columbia Press, 2012.

– *When Good Drugs Go Bad: Opium, Medicine, and the Origins of Canada's Drug Laws*. Vancouver, BC: University of British Columbia Press, 2015.

Marantz, Paul, Elizabeth Bird, and Michael Alderman. "A Call for a Higher Standards of Evidence for Dietary Guidelines." *American Journal of Preventive Medicine* 34, no. 3 (2008): 234–40.

Markle, Gerald E., and James C. Peterson. *Politics, Science, and Cancer: The Laetrile Phenomenon*. Boulder, CO: Westview Press, 1980.

Marquis, Greg. "From Beverage to Drug: Alcohol and Other Drugs in 1960s and 1970s Canada." *Journal of Canadian Studies* 39, no. 2 (2005): 57–79.

Martel, Marcel. *Not This Time: Canadians, Public Policy, and the Marijuana Question, 1961–1975*. Toronto: University of Toronto Press, 2011.

Mattingly, Patricia, and Stephanie T. Conley. "The Medical Prescription of Heroin for Terminal Cancer Patients." *Lawyer's Medical Journal* 9, no. 3 (1981): 337–54.

May, Gary. *Bending toward Justice: The Voting Rights Act and the Transformation of American Democracy*. New York: Basic Books, 2013.

McAllister, William. *Drug Diplomacy in the Twentieth Century*. New York: Routledge, 1999.

McCarthy, Michael. "Epinephrine Pen Maker Offers Discount after Alleged Price Hiking." *British Medical Journal* 354 (2016): i4730.

McGirr, Lisa. *The War on Alcohol: Prohibition and the Rise of the American State*. New York: W.W. Norton, 2016.

McWilliams, John C. "Unsung Partner against Crime: Harry J. Anslinger and the Federal Bureau of Narcotics, 1930–1962." *The Pennsylvania Magazine of History and Biography* 113, no. 2 (1989): 207–36.

Michaels, David. "Manufactured Uncertainty: Protecting Public Health in the Age of Contested Science and Product Defense." *Annals of the New York Academy of Sciences* 1076 (2006): 149–62.

Milkis, Sidney M., and Jerome M. Mileur, eds. *The Great Society and the High Tide of Liberalism*. Boston, MA: University of Massachusetts Press, 2005.

Miller, Henry I., and David R. Henderson. "The FDA's Risky Risk-Aversion." *Policy Review* 145 (2007): 3–27.

Miller, Richard J. "The Cannabis Conundrum." *Proceedings of the National Academy of Sciences of the United States of America* 110, no. 43 (2013): 17165.

Mills, James H. *Cannabis Britannica: Empire, Trade, and Prohibition 1800–1928*. Oxford, UK: Oxford University Press, 2005.

– *Cannabis Nation: Control and Consumption in Britain, 1928–2008*.
  Oxford, UK: Oxford University Press, 2013.
Mills, John A. "Lessons from the Periphery: Psychiatry in Saskatchewan,
  Canada, 1944–1968." *History of Psychiatry* 18, no. 2 (2007): 179–201.
Moertel, C.G. "A Trial of Laetrile Now." *New England Journal of
  Medicine* 298, no. 4 (1978): 218–19.
Mold, Alex. *Heroin: The Treatment of Addiction in Twentieth-Century
  Britain*. Champaign, IL: Northern Illinois University Press, 2008.
Montigny, Ed, ed. *The Real Dope: Social, Legal, and Historical
  Perspectives on the Regulation of Drugs in Canada*. Toronto: University
  of Toronto Press, 2011.
Morgan, John. *Phenylpropanolamine: A Critical Analysis of Adverse
  Reactions and Overdosage*. Englewood, NJ: Jack K. Burgess Inc., 1986.
Morgan, John P., and Frank R. Funderburk. "Phenylpropanolamine and
  Blood Pressure: A Review of Prospective Studies." *American Journal of
  Clinical Nutrition* 55 (1992): 206S–10S.
Morris, Kelly. "Research on Psychedelics Moves Into the Mainstream."
  The Lancet 361, no. 9623 (2008): 1491–2.
Moss, Ralph W. *The Cancer Industry*. New York: Equinox Press, 1980.
Musto, David. *The American Disease: Origins of Narcotic Control*. New
  York: Oxford University Press, 2003.
– ed. *One Hundred Years of Heroin*. New York: Praeger, 2002.
Musto, David, and Pamela Korsmeyer. *The Quest for Drug Control:
  Politics and Federal Policy in a Period of Increasing Substance Abuse,
  1963–1981*. New Haven, CT: Yale University Press, 2002.
National Cancer Institute. "Clinical Study of Laetrile in Cancer Patients,
  Investigators' Report: A Summary." Bethesda, MD: NCI, 30 April 1981.
National Library of Medicine. "Ketamine." *Toxnet: Toxicology Data
  Network*. https://toxnet.nlm.nih.gov/cgibin/sis/search/a?dbs+hsdb:@
  term+@DOCNO+2180 (accessed 18 October 2016).
Newman, Laura. "Elisabeth Kubler-Ross: Psychiatrist and Pioneer of the
  Death-and-Dying Movement." *British Medical Journal* 329, no. 7466
  (2004): 627.
NHS Health Scotland. "NHS Health Scotland Position Statement on
  E-cigarettes 2015." 30 November 2015. http://www.healthscotland.
  com/documents/24383.aspx.
Nightingale, Stuart L. "Laetrile: The Regulatory Challenge of an Unproven
  Remedy." *Public Health Reports* 99, no. 4 (1984): 333–8.

Nunn, Kenneth. "Race, Crime and the Pool of Surplus Criminality: Or Why the 'War on Drugs' was a 'War on Blacks.'" *Journal of Gender, Race & Justice* 6 (2002): 381–445.

"Nurses' Drug Alert: Diet Pills and Stroke." *American Journal of Nursing* 87, no. 8 (1987): 1070.

Nutt, David. *Drugs without the Hot Air: Minimizing the Harms of Legal and Illegal* Drugs. Cambridge: UIT Cambridge Ltd, 2012.

Offit, Paul. *Autism's False Prophets: Bad Science, Risky Medicine, and the Search for a Cure*. New York: Columbia University Press, 2010.

– *Deadly Choices: How the Anti-Vaccine Movement Threatens Us All*. New York: Basic Books, 2010.

Oliver, Eric. *Fat Politics: The Real Story behind America's Obesity Epidemic*. New York: Oxford University Press, 2006.

Olson, Mary. "Substitution in Regulatory Agencies: FDA Enforcement Alternatives." *Journal of Law, Economics and Organization* 12, no. 2 (1996): 376–407.

Oram, Matthew. "Efficacy and Enlightenment: LSD Psychotherapy and the Drug Amendments of 1962." *Journal of the History of Medicine and Allied Sciences* 69, no. 2 (2014): 221–50.

Osmond, Humphry. "A Review of the Clinical Effects of Psychotomimetic Agents." *Annals of the New York Academy of Sciences* 66, no. 3 (1957): 418–34.

Page, Jonathan, and Mark Ware. "Perspective: Close the Knowledge Gap." *Nature* 525, no. 7570 (2015): S9.

Pajevic, I., et al. "Do Cannabis and Cannabinoids Have a Psychofarmalogically Therapeutic Effect?" *European Psychiatry* 30, no. 1 (2015): 1068.

Paradis, Lenora Finn, and Scott B. Cummings. "The Evolution of Hospice in America toward Organizational Homogeneity." *Journal of Health and Social Behavior* 27, no. 4 (1986): 370–86.

Park, Roberta J. "Historical Reflections on Diet, Exercise, and Obesity: The Recurring Need to 'Put Words into Action.'" *Canadian Bulletin for Medical History* 28, no. 2 (2011): 383–401.

Patterson, James T. *The Dread Disease: Cancer and Modern American Culture*. Cambridge, MA: Harvard University Press, 1989.

PDQ® Integrative, Alternative, and Complementary Therapies Editorial Board. "PDQ Laetrile/Amygdalin." Bethesda, MD: National Cancer Institute, 2012. https://www.cancer.gov/about-cancer/treatment/cam/hp/laetrile-pdq (accessed 11 October 2016).

Peasley, Edgar. "For Patients Having Coma Shock Therapy." *The American Journal of Nursing* 49, no. 10 (1949): 623–6.

Pembleton, Matthew R. *Containing Addiction: The Federal Bureau of Narcotics and the Origins of America's Global Drug War.* Boston, MA: University of Massachusetts Press, 2017.

Peters, Lulu Hunt. *Diet and Health with Key to the Calories.* New York: The Reilly and Lee Co., 1925.

Pieters, Toine, and Stephen Snelders. "From King Kong Pills to Mother's Little Helpers – Career Cycles of Two Families of Psychotropic Drugs: The Barbiturates and Benzodiazepines." *Canadian Bulletin of Medical History* 24, no. 1 (2007): 93–112.

Pines, Wayne, ed. FDA: *A Century of Consumer Protection.* Washington, DC: Food and Drug Law Institute, 2006.

Pollan, Michael. *In Defense of Food: An Eater's Manifesto.* New York: Penguin, 2008.

Porath-Waller, A.J., J.E. Brown, A.P. Frigon, and H. Clark. *What Canadian Youth Think about Cannabis.* Ottawa: Canadian Centre on Substance Abuse, 2013. http://www.ccsa.ca/Resource%20Library/CCSA-What-Canadian-Youth-Think-about-Cannabis-2013-en.pdf (accessed 18 January 2017).

Public Citizen's Congress Watch. "The Other Drug War 2003: Drug Companies Deploy an Army of 675 Lobbyists to Protect Profits." 2004. http://www.citizen.org/documents/Other_Drug_War2003.pdf (accessed 17 October 2016).

Quon, Nicole. "Decisions at Scientific Agencies: How Do the NIH and FDA Balance Expert Opinions, Changing Agendas, and Political Pressure?" PhD diss. New Haven, CT: Yale University, 2007.

Radin, Paul. *The Trickster: A Study in American Indian Mythology.* New York: Schocken Press, 1987.

Rasmussen, Keith G., et al. "Serial Infusions of Low-Dose Ketamine for Major Depression." *Journal of Psychopharmacology* 27, no. 5 (2013): 444–50.

Reagan, Ronald, Kiron K. Skinner, Annelise Anderson, et al. *Reagan, in His Own Hand: The Writings of Ronald Reagan That Reveal His Revolutionary Vision for America.* New York: Touchstone Book, 2001.

Rees, Alan M. "Characteristics, Content, and Significance of the Popular Health Periodicals Literature." *Bulletin of the Medical Libraries Association* 75, no. 4 (1987): 317–22.

Relman, Arnold S. "Laetrilomania – Again." *New England Journal of Medicine* 298, no. 4 (1978): 215–16.

– "Closing the Books on Laetrile (Editorial)." *New England Journal of Medicine* 306, no. 4 (1982): 236.

Richardson, John, and Patricia Griffin. *Laetrile Case Histories: The Richardson Cancer Clinic Experience.* New York: Bantam Books, 1977.

Richert, Lucas. "Pills, Policy Making and Perceptions: Inside the FDA during the 'Reagan Revolution,' 1981–1982." *Canadian Review of American Studies* 39, no. 1 (2009): 41–63.

– "Surveying the Seventies: Something's Still Happening." *Canadian Journal of History* 46, no. 3 (2011): 649–54.

– *Conservatism, Consumer Choice, and the Food and Drug Administration during the Reagan Era: A Prescription for Scandal.* Lanham, MD: Lexington Books, 2014.

– "'Therapy Means Political Change, Not Peanut Butter': American Radical Psychiatry, 1968–1975." *Social History of Medicine* 24, no. 1 (2014): 104–21.

– "Heroin in the Hospice: Opioids and End-of-Life Discussions in the 1980s." *Canadian Medical Association Journal* 189 (2 October 2017): E1231–2.

Rizzolatti, Giamcomo, Cinzia Di Dio, and Emiliano Macaluso. "The Golden Beauty: Brain Response to Classical and Renaissance Sculptures." *Plos One* 2, no. 11 (2007): e1201. doi:10.1371/journal.pone.0001201.

Room, Robin. "Cannabis Legalization and Public Health: Legal Niceties, Commercialization and Countercultures." *Addiction* 109, no. 3 (2014): 358–9.

Rorabaugh, William. *Prohibition: A Concise History.* New York: Oxford University Press, 2018.

Rosenberg, Charles. "Pathologies of Progress: The Idea of Civilization at Risk." *Bulletin of the History of Medicine* 72, no. 4 (1998): 714–30.

Rotunda, Michele. "Savages to the Left of Me, Neurasthenics to the Right, Stuck in the Middle with You: Inebriety and Human Nature in American Society, 1855–1900." *Canadian Bulletin of Medical History* 24, no. 1 (2007): 49–65.

Rowe, Jonathan, and Judith Silverstein. "The GDP Myth: Why 'Growth' Isn't Always a Good Thing." *The Washington Monthly* 31, no. 3 (1999): 17–21.

Rucker, James J.H. "Views and Reviews." *British Medical Journal* 350 (26 May 2015). doi:https://doi.org/10.1136/bmj.h2902.

Saatsoglou, Paul. "Pharmaceutical Reimportation: Magnitude, Trends, and Consumers." *Managed Care* 13, no. 3 (2004): 7–9.

Sadowsky, Jonathan. *Electroconvulsive Therapy in America: The Anatomy of a Medical Controversy*. New York: Routledge, 2017.

Scarry, Elaine. *The Body in Pain: The Making and Unmaking of the World*. Oxford, UK: Oxford University Press, 1987.

Schatzberg, Alan F. "A Word to the Wise about Ketamine." *American Journal of Psychiatry* 171, no. 3 (2014): 262–4.

Schneider, Eric. *Smack: Heroin and the American City*. Philadelphia, PA: University of Pennsylvania Press, 2008.

Schrag, Peter. "A Quagmire for Our Time: The War on Drugs." *Journal of Public Health Policy* 23, no. 3 (2002): 286–98.

Schulman, Bruce. *The Seventies: The Great Shift in American Culture, Society, and Politics*. New York: Da Capo Press, 2001.

Schulman, Bruce, and Julian Zelizer, eds. *Rightward Bound: Making American Conservative in the 1970s*. Cambridge, MA: University of Massachusetts Press, 2008.

Schwantes, Carlos A. *In Mountain Shadows: A History of Idaho*. Lincoln: University of Nebraska Press, 1991.

Schwartz, Hillel. *Never Satisfied: A Cultural History of Diets, Fantasies and Fat*. New York: Free Press, 1986.

Scott, John F., and E.M. Sellers. *Cancer Pain, A Monograph on the Management of Cancer Pain: A Report of the Expert Advisory Committee on the Management of Severe Chronic Pain in Cancer Patients*. Ottawa: Health and Welfare Canada, 1984.

Scroop, Daniel. "A Faded Passion? Estes Kefauver and the Senate Subcommittee on Antitrust and Monopoly." *Business and Economic History On-Line* 5 (2007): 1–17.

Sessa, Ben. *The Psychedelic Renaissance: Reassessing the Role of Psychedelic Drugs in 21st Century Psychiatry and Society*. London: Muswell Hill Press, 2012.

– "Turn On and Tune In to Evidence-Based Psychedelic Research." *The Lancet Psychiatry* 2, no. 1 (2015): 10–12.

Shepherd, Marv. "Drug Importation and Safety of Drugs Obtained from Canada." *Annals of Pharmacotherapy* 41, no. 7–8 (2007): 1288–91.

Shilts, Randy. *And the Band Played On: Politics, People, and the AIDS Epidemic*. New York: St Martin's Press, 2007.

Shrubb, Richard. "The Magical Mystery Cure." *Therapy Today* 24, no. 4 (2013): 10.

Sidney, Stephen. "Comparing Cannabis with Tobacco – Again: Link between Cannabis and Mortality Is Still Not Established." *BMJ: British Medical Journal* 327, no. 7416 (2003): 635–6.

Siff, Stephen. *Acid Hype: American News Media and the Psychedelic Experience.* Urbana: University of Illinois Press, 2015.

Sismondo, Christine. *America Walks into a Bar: A Spirited History of Taverns and Saloons, Speakeasies and Grog Shops.* New York: Oxford University Press, 2011.

Skinner, Brent. "Price Controls, Patents, and Cross-Border Internet Pharmacies: Risks to Canada's Drug Supply and International Trading Relations." *The Fraser Institute: Critical Issues Bulletin* (2006): 1–36.

Skinner, Brett J. "Prescription Piracy: The Black Market in Foreign Drugs Will Not Reduce U.S. Healthcare Costs." In *What States Can Do to Reform Health Care: A Free-Market Primer*, edited by John R. Graham. San Francisco, CA: Pacific Research Institute, 2006.

Small, Dan, and Ernest Drucker. "Policy Makers Ignoring Science and Scientists Ignoring Policy: The Medical Ethical Challenges of Heroin Treatment." *Harm Reduction Journal* 3 (2006): 16.

Smith, Andrew F. *Eating History: Thirty Turning Points in the Making of American Cuisine.* New York: Columbia University Press, 2009.

Smith, David E., Glen Raswyck, and Leigh Dickerson. "From Hofmann to the Haight Ashbury, and into the Future: The Past and Present of Lysergic Acid Diethlyamide." *Journal of Psychoactive Drugs* 46, no. 1 (2014): 3–10.

Smith, Matthew. *Hyperactive: The Controversial History of ADHD.* London: Reaktion Books, 2012.

Snelders, Stephen, Charles Kaplan, and Toine Pieters. "On Cannabis, Chloral Hydrate, and Career Cycles of Psychotropic Drugs in Medicine." *Bulletin for Medical History* 80, no. 1 (2006): 95–114.

Spithoff, Sheryl, Brian Emerson, and Andrea Spithoff. "Cannabis Legalization: Adhering to Public Health Best Practice." *Canadian Medical Association Journal* 187, no. 16 (2015): 1211–16.

Stearns, Peter. *Fat History: Bodies and Beauty in the Modern West.* New York: New York University Press, 2002.

Stein, Judith. *Pivotal Decade: How the United States Traded Factories for Finance in the Seventies.* New Haven, CT: Yale University Press, 2010.

Stevens, Jay. *Storming Heaven: LSD and the American Dream.* New York: Grove Press, 1987.

Stogner, David, et al., eds. *Synthetic and Novel Drugs: Emerging Issues, Legal Policy and Public Health.* Boca Raton, FL: CRC Press, 2017.

Stoll, S.M. "Why Not Heroin? The Controversy Surrounding the Legalization of Heroin for Therapeutic Purposes." *Journal of Contemporary Health Policy and Law* 1 (1985): 173–94.

Sun, Marjorie. "Laetrile Brush Fire Is Out, Scientists Hope." *Science* 212, no. 4496 (1981): 758–9.

– "Heroin, Morphine Found Comparable as Pain-Killer." *Science* 216, no. 4543 (1982): 277.

Szasz, Thomas. *Our Right to Drugs: The Case for a Free Market.* Syracuse, NY: Syracuse University Press, 1996.

Sznitman, Sharol R., and Yuval Zolotov. "Cannabis for Therapeutic Purposes and Public Health and Safety: A Systematic and Critical Review." *International Journal of Drug Policy* 26, no. 1 (2015): 20–9.

Talbott, John A. "Fifty Years of Psychiatric Services: Changes in Treatments of Chronically Ill Patients." In *Review of Psychiatry Volume 13*, edited by John M. Oldham and Michelle B. Riba. Washington, DC: American Psychiatric Press, 1994.

Thernstrom, Melanie. *The Pain Chronicles: Cures, Myths, Mysteries; Prayers, Diaries, Brain Scans, Healing and the Science of Suffering.* New York: Picador, 2011.

Thompson, M. Guy. *The Legacy of R.D. Laing: An Appraisal of His Contemporary Relevance.* New York: Routledge, 2015.

Tobbell, Dominique. "'Who's Winning the Human Race?' Cold War as Pharmaceutical Political Strategy." *Journal of the History of Medicine and Allied Sciences* 64, no. 4 (2009): 429–73.

Tomes, Nancy. "Merchants of Health: Medicine and Consumer Culture in the United States, 1900–1940." *The Journal of American History* 88, no. 2 (2001): 519–47.

Torrens, Paul, ed. *Hospice Program and Public Policy.* Chicago, IL: American Hospital Publishing, 1985.

Trebach, Arnold. *The Great Drug War: And Rational Proposals to Turn the Tide.* New York: Macmillan Publishing, 1987.

Troetel, Barbara Resnick. "Three Part Disharmony: The Transformation of the Food and Drug Administration in the 1970s." PhD diss. New York: City University of New York, 1996.

Twycross, R.G. "Stumbling Blocks in the Study of Diamorphine." *Postgraduate Medical Journal* 49 (1973): 309–13.

– "Clinical Experience with Diamorphine in Advanced Malignant Disease." *International Journal of Clinical Pharmacology, Therapy, and Toxicology* 9, no. 3 (1974): 184–98.

– "Choice of Strong Analgesic in Terminal Cancer: Diamorphine or Morphine?" *Pain* 3, no. 2 (1977): 93–104.

Uchtenhagen, Ambros. "Some Critical Issues in Cannabis Policy Reform." *Addiction* 109, no. 3 (2014): 356–8.

Vester, Katharina. "Regime Change: Gender, Class, and the Invention of Dieting in Post-Bellum America." *Journal of Social History* 44, no. 1 (2010): 39–70.

Vollenweider, Franz X., and Michael Kometer. "The Neurobiology of Psychedelic Drugs: Implications for the Treatment of Mood Disorders." *Nature Reviews Neuroscience* 11, no. 9 (2010): 642–51.

Wailoo, Keith. *Pain: A Political History*. Baltimore, MD: Johns Hopkins University Press, 2014.

Walker, Ken. "How a Medical Journalist Helped to Legalize Heroin in Canada." *Journal of Drug Issues* 21, no. 1 (1991): 141–6.

Wall, Patrick. *Pain: The Science of Suffering*. New York: Columbia University Press, 2002.

Walsh, John. "Laetrile Tops FDA's Most Unwanted List." *Science* 199, no. 4325 (1978): 158–9.

Ward, Christopher. "Economic Policy Implications of Reimportation: A Canadian Perspective." *Managed Care* 13, no. 3 (2004): 17–20.

Ware, Mark, et al. "Smoked Cannabis for Chronic Neuropathic Pain: A Randomized Controlled Trial." *Canadian Medical Association Journal* 182, no. 14 (2010): E694–701.

– "Cannabis for the Management of Pain: Assessment of Safety Study (COMPASS)." *The Journal of Pain* 16, no. 12 (2015): 1233–42.

Ware, Mark, and Julie Desroches. "Medical Cannabis and Pain." *Pain: Clinical Updates* 22, no. 3 (2014): 1–7.

Warsh, Cheryl Krasnick, ed. *Gender, Health, and Popular Culture: Historical Perspectives*. Waterloo, ON: Wilfrid Laurier University Press, 2011.

Wasson, Robert Gordon. *Soma: Divine Mushroom of Immortality*. New York: Harcourt, 1972.

Watters, Ethan. *Crazy Like Us: The Globalization of the American Psyche*. New York: Free Press, 2010.

Wilkinson, Samuel T., Mesut Toprak, Mason S. Turner, et al. "A Survey of the Clinical, Off-Label Use of Ketamine as a Treatment for Psychiatric Disorders." *American Journal of Psychiatry* 174, no. 7 (2017): 695–6.

Wilson, James Q., Mark H. Moore, and I. David Wheat. "The Problem of Heroin." *The Public Interest* 29 (1972): 3–28.

Winkler, Petr, and Ladislav Csémy. "Self-Experimentations with Psychedelics among Mental Health Professionals: LSD in the Former Czechoslovakia." *Journal of Psychoactive Drugs* 46, no. 1 (2014): 11–19.

World Health Organization. "WHO Recommends against International Control of Ketamine." December 2015. http://www.who.int/medicines/access/controlled-substances/recommends_against_ick/en/ (accessed 20 January 2017).

Yen, M., and M.B. Ewald. "Toxicity of Weight Loss Agents." *Journal of Medical Toxicology* 8, no. 2 (2012): 142–52.

Young, James Harvey. *American Health Quackery: Collected Essays of James Harvey Young*. Princeton, NJ: Princeton University Press, 1992.

– *The Medical Messiahs: A Social History of Medical Quackery in 20th Century America*. Princeton, NJ: Princeton University Press, 1992.

Zarate, Carlos, Jaskaram B. Singh, Paul Carlson, et al. "A Randomized Trial of an N-methyl-D-asparate Antagonist in Treatment-Resistant Major Depression." *Archives of General Psychiatry* 63, no. 8 (2006): 856–64.

Zelizer, Julian. *The Fierce Urgency of Now: Lyndon Johnson, Congress, and the Battle for the Great Society*. New York: Penguin Press, 2015.

INDEX